WHEN FAITH & LOVE CONFRONT CANCER

A Journey Through the Battlefield
of Cancer and How We Survived

EVELYN KORMONDY

Praise for *When Faith & Love Confront Cancer*

"This remarkable love story of two cancer survivors will strengthen your faith and renew hope to anyone diagnosed with cancer or a serious illness. It's such an incredible message of God's favor and healing through unwavering faith and prayer. The author's details and accounts are awe-inspiring and divine! This book will leave you feeling deeply connected to God's Word and encouraged!"

Amber Canterbury, Wife and Mother

"An inspiring story of luck, love, faith, and divine intervention overcoming health challenges."

Robert Lee, Attorney

"Here is an engaging, straightforward, and honest story about a couple who have endured the ravages of cancer multiple times. It revolves around God, their faith in Him, and their desire to see His will done. Whether you are facing difficult circumstances or not, this book is an encouragement to live your life for God. I highly recommend it."

Steve Baumgartner, Bible Study Leader

"Evelyn Kormondy shares with courageous honesty the tough experiences that have shaped her and Bob's journey together and with Christ. Her genuine authenticity and vulnerable transparency are refreshing and inspirational to those struggling through the unpredictable storms of life. As an Army Chaplain, I will use this invaluable tool as a blueprint in guiding soldiers as they face troubling circumstances. It is possible to live a fulfilling life of faith NO MATTER WHAT!"

CH (CPT) Shane Withrow, Chaplain US ARMY

Table of Contents

Introduction I

Chapter 1:   Table Twenty-One 1

Chapter 2:   He's Back!... 9

Chapter 3:   A Long Time Coming......................... 17

Chapter 4:   "I Do!"...27

Chapter 5:   Living The Dream............................. 32

Chapter 6:   What's Wrong? 37

Chapter 7:   Australia, Here We Come! 44

Chapter 8:   The Diagnosis 48

Chapter 9:   Four Months To Live...........................55

Chapter 10:   Tick Tock, Tick Tock......................... 64

Chapter 11:   Don't Leave...................................74

Chapter 12:   The Kormondy Medical Center 82

Chapter 13:   Who Knew About The Teeth? 91

Chapter 14:   The Plan To Survive 95

Chapter 15:   Financial Hardship...........................106

Chapter 16:   The Mask Of Precision 110

Chapter 17:   God's Gift Of A Second Chance.......... 118

Chapter 18:   Feeding The Feeding Tube.................123

Chapter 19:   A Shot In The Arm........................... 131

Chapter 20:   A Child's Faith 136

Chapter 21:   The Last Time....................................142

Chapter 22:   Life Without Radiation 147

Chapter 23:   Returning To His Passion 151

Chapter 24:   Imminent Foreclosure....................... 157

Chapter 25:   No More Feeding Tube! 167

Chapter 26:   Defying The Odds............................ 176

Chapter 27:   Was That A Lump?............................ 184

Chapter 28:   Keeping Secrets 194

Chapter 29:   I Don't Belong Here! 201

Chapter 30:   A More-Than-Likely Diagnosis......... 208

Chapter 31 :   Why? Why? Why? 214

Chapter 32:   Definitely Not A Quick Fix 222

Chapter 33:   Reporting For Duty 228

Chapter 34:   The Red Devil 237

Chapter 35:   The Chemo Fog............................... 243

Chapter 36:   The Loss Of Losing My Hair 249

Chapter 37:   Lake Tahoe, Here We Come Again! .. 256

Chapter 38:   Taking Back My Power...................... 265

Chapter 39:   Pink Tears.....................................275

Chapter 40:   The Intensity Intensifies 281

Chapter 41:   You Are Stronger Than Cancer 289

Chapter 42:   Team Kormondy................................297

Chapter 43:   Preparing To Face The Giant 302

Chapter 44:   We've Got This! 310

Chapter 45:   Just When You Think It's Over.......... 320

Chapter 46: Miss Camo And Pearls 327

Chapter 47: The Last Chemo Treatment 334

Chapter 48: My First Radiation Treatment 340

Chapter 49: The Slow Burn 348

Chapter 50: The Final Time 355

Chapter 51: Reconstruction Surgery #1................ 364

Chapter 52: They're Not Right! 376

Chapter 53: Reconstruction Surgery #2 382

Chapter 54: Three Strikes, And You're Out! 385

Chapter 55: An Answer To Prayer 393

Conclusion 402

Inspirational Poems 407

Inspirational Scriptures 421

Helpful Hints 425

About The Author: Evelyn Kormondy 427

*I dedicate this book to God
and to my husband, Bob Kormondy.*

Oh Dear Lord
Three things I pray
To see thee more clearly
Love thee more dearly
Follow thee more nearly
Day by day.

(These words helped me get through
each day during my battle with cancer.)

Disclaimer

This book is a memoir, a book of memories. It reflects my present recollections of experiences over time, and I have made every effort to recreate this story as accurately as possible.

The names and characteristics of everyone in this book, except for family members, Lori McSwain, Christian Schwartzer, Sabrena and Brad Reed, Joseph E. Miller, Motswedi, Liz, Aidan, and Kathy McCoy, have been changed to respect their privacy. In addition, some events have been compressed, and some dialogue has been recreated.

All poems in this book written by Peggy Dailey were printed with permission by Peggy Daily.

The purpose of this book is to enlighten and entertain. Neither I nor the publisher provide medical advice, and we have no knowledge of your specific needs. If you need any medical advice, please contact your doctor directly. Neither I nor the publisher have liability nor responsibility to any person or entity with respect to any loss or damage caused, or alleged to have been caused, directly or indirectly, by the information contained in this book.

Acknowledgements

First and foremost, I thank God for His unending love.

Next, I thank my husband Bob for his love and support.

Thank you to my parents, Jack and Patricia Ashcroft, for always believing in me.

Thanks to Michelle, Charlene, and Kristy for keeping me laughing when I wanted to cry.

Thanks to my family and their much-needed love and support.

Thank you to my dear friend Kathy McCoy and my sister Shirley Glasgow for being there during both good and awful times.

A heartfelt thank you goes to Sherrie Clark for her guidance with this book.

I would be remiss if I didn't thank Laurie McSwain, a friend I met along the way who guided me through the journey. I love you. Keep fighting the fight, and thank you for always helping others.

Bryan my dear friend continue fighting the fight you've got this.

Love to Mary D. for being an amazingly strong woman during the fight.

Janet, I love you. You have got this!

And thank you to my church family for all your prayers, love, and support.

Introduction

One couple with *four* cancer diagnoses and *two* people miraculously alive to tell the story!

To know our secret is to understand Bob's and my journey, one that you'll embark upon within these pages. But this isn't a book about cancer. Instead, it's a love story of two people who, when attacked by a faceless yet strong enemy, prove that their love and their God are much stronger.

So follow me as I take you on a journey behind the mysterious veil of cancer and expose what its victims go through, and most importantly, how they survive. It involves battles, with the greatest taking place beyond medical test results and treatments.

But I won't leave you hanging. I'll show you how we fought back—and won—after we were yanked onto the battlefield time and again for our lives.

The Battle

Cancer had flirted with both Bob and me years earlier. We had been diagnosed with different types of cancer, but we had survived; in fact, we had put them behind us and moved on. But cancer hadn't. It came back after us, stepping up its tactics exponentially.

It tried its best to take down Bob with cancer so aggressive that the doctors gave him only four months to live. Although cancer is not a respecter of persons, to me, it was very personal. No way was it taking my husband, the love of my life! The warrior in me reared up. With my weapons of warfare sharpened and me suited up in armor, I came out swinging my sword, His Word, while holding up my shield of faith to cover my husband. As a result, Jesus was right there with me, and cancer had to retreat.

Oh, but cancer was not done with the Kormondys. Before we had a chance to catch our breath from our last victory, cancer came at me with a vengeance. I was diagnosed with an aggressive form of cancer, different from Bob's but just as deadly.

Battle-weary with chinks in my armor and now too weak to stand, I stayed on my knees as Bob picked up the sword. The Spirit of God joined forces with us. Cancer fought back hard, but it proved to be no match!

Its problem—underestimating a powerful God!

The Purpose of This Book

Writing this book was a calling. Our story is unique because we had fought cancer—and won—four times! But sadly, a total of 1.9 million new cancer cases are expected in 2022.[1]

When someone is told they have cancer, they most likely get overwhelmed with fear, and a lot of that fear comes from the unknown—*What does this look like? What will I go through? Will I live or die?* We understand.

As a result, I wanted to shine a light on some of those unknowns to empower you should you or a loved one get diagnosed with cancer. You can have an idea of what to expect, and elements of surprise are no longer so surprising. Knowledge is power.

But for those who are in the throes of cancer, I wanted to encourage you through statistics. According

---

1 ACS Medical Content and News Staff, "Risk of Dying for Cancer Continues to Drop at an Accelerated Pace," American Cancer Society, January 12, 2022, accessed February 9, 2022, https://www.cancer.org/latest-news/facts-and-figures-2022.html.

to the American Cancer Society, "The risk of dying from cancer in the United States has decreased over the past 28 years."[2] Still, cancer is scary, so I wanted to also inspire you through Bob's and my many battles. I hope our story helps you realize that it is possible to overcome the travesty of what cancer does. You can overcome anything that cancer throws at you with the strength and love of God, family, and friends to help you along the way.

If you don't have family and friends, don't worry. Your biggest and strongest ally is God. You will always have Him no matter how far away from Him you think you are. He had always been there for you—always will be—and He has also given you the same weapons He gave to Bob and me. He's just waiting on you to pick them up and use them.

Through our story, I'll show you how.

YOU ARE STRONGER THAN CANCER

All along the way of our journey, we reminded each other that we were stronger than cancer. These weren't nice or empty words, but they gave us the wherewithal

---

2   Ibid.

to stand, although sometimes on shaky legs. And if nothing else, we simply stood and let God fight this battle for us.

And He did!

These pages reveal a testimony that proves nothing is too big for our God. When cancer swooped in to destroy us, three pairs of footprints became one as God picked us up and carried us. So, never ever give up, even when it looks dismal.

With God, ALL things are possible, and that includes life!

– 1 –

Table Twenty-One?

My marriage to Bob was perfect. I knew he was the one from the first moment I spoke to him.

At that time, I had been working for my father's company, Ashcroft's Creative Cabinets, as an interior designer, office manager, and bookkeeper. But on the weekends, I helped out my friend Rose at Alonzo's Italian Restaurant where she was the manager. It was small, family-run and operated, and everyone there felt like family, from the owner to the cooks to all the customers, most of whom were regulars. As the hostess, I got to meet and greet them and walk them to their tables.

Not only did the people make Alonzo's my favorite restaurant, but I also loved its quaint and romantic atmosphere accentuated by soft lighting—the ideal setting for meeting the man of your dreams.

On Saturday evening, November 25, 1995, I happened to be at the right place at the right time—working at Alonzo's. While standing by the bar, a tall, slim man with short dark hair came in alone. I had never seen him before, and I was definitely impressed.

The restaurant's owner, Peter, was working the bar behind me. He knew most of the patrons, or at least he knew about them.

"Hey, Peter, do you know the gentleman who just walked in?" I asked over my shoulder without taking my eyes off our new customer.

"Yeah, that's Bob. He's been in here before. Works for NBC Sports. Maybe he's in town because of the Jags game tomorrow. Seems like a really nice guy."

Hmm. Well, that increased my intrigue. I loved sports, especially football, and I was a big fan of our hometown NFL football team, the Jacksonville Jaguars.

Smiling, I walked up to the handsome newcomer and found myself staring into the most beautiful blue eyes I had ever seen. I finally managed to utter, "Welcome to Alonzo's. Smoking or nonsmoking?"

"Nonsmoking," he replied, returning my smile . . . and stare.

After tearing my eyes away from him, I thought, *So far, so good. He doesn't smoke.* He just scored one point on my self-created attraction system for men.

Glancing down at his right hand, I didn't see a ring either. Another point. Within a couple of seconds, he had gotten himself up to two points. Very impressive to me.

Continuing to smile at him, I said, "Follow me" and then turned with a little sashay.

"Absolutely!" One word, but it was said with such a sexy voice that it caused the hair on the back of my neck to stand straight up.

Oh my goodness, I thought, *I am in trouble.*

Once we arrived at his booth (much too soon, I may add), and he sat down, I gave him a menu. "Your server will be with you soon," I informed him.

The server for this table was gathering drinks at the bar for other customers. I rushed over to her and leaned close to her ear. "Marsha, do you mind if I take table twenty-one? Just this time?"

Her eyes darted to table twenty-one and then back at me. She furrowed her eyebrows in confusion. "But you're not a server, Evelyn. You're a hostess."

I glanced at the table and back at her with a shrug and a smile. "That's okay. I've got this."

Her eyes followed mine. Then she slowly nodded in understanding as a smile spread across her face. "Sure. He's all yours, but I want the tip."

"Deal," I agreed, curious about her statement "He's all yours."

Turning back to the dining room, I thought, *Okay, Evelyn, time to give the change of plans to the handsome man.*

As I approached his table, he looked up at me with those blue eyes that I knew I could easily get lost in. "Hey, do you know where my server is?" he asked.

"Your server's busy right now, so I'll be able to help you." It was the truth; she was busy delivering those drinks to another table.

He smiled, and I could almost see his body relaxing. "I'd like to go ahead and place my order then."

"Sure," I responded. "What can I get for you?"

"I'd like the manicotti."

I realized I didn't have anything to write his order on. But how hard was it to remember manicotti?

"Manicotti," I confirmed.

He nodded while his eyes lingered on mine.

I finally forced myself to leave and give the order to

the kitchen. "By the way," I started my announcement just loud enough for the kitchen staff to hear, "I'm gonna take table twenty-one."

Their perplexed faces told me that I should scurry myself out of there before they could ask me any questions.

I returned to the podium up front to join my friend Rose and stood next to her.

"Rose, that's the man for me," I proclaimed with a huge grin on my face. "The one at table twenty-one. I'm going to marry him."

I was in my thirties and had remained single by choice. I had rather be alone than marry someone who wasn't the right person for the sake of fitting in with my married friends. But now, and for the first time in my life, I started feeling what I had only heard others describe—butterflies fluttering around in my stomach.

Rose turned and stared at me for a moment as if contemplating my announcement. "How do you know that, Evelyn?"

I shrugged. "It's a feeling. I just know he's the one. I know that when I greeted him at the door, he had the most amazing smile and seemed so warm and kind.

I know that when I spoke with him, he seemed very intelligent and fun, and he was able to draw me into whatever he said. I know that when I'm around him, I already feel really comfortable. Yep, he's the one for me, the man I'm marrying. I just know it."

She smiled and rolled her eyes. "Evelyn, do you even know his name?"

"As a matter of fact, I do," I answered with a tilt of my chin in mocked defiance. "It's Bob, and he works for NBC Sports. Now if you don't mind, I've got work to do."

Rose chuckled. "Um-hum. I'm sure you do."

I sauntered over to the bar. "Peter, since we're not that busy, you're gonna see me over at table twenty-one a lot because I like that guy."

He laughed. "Okay, but keep an eye on the other tables and the door." Peter was a wonderful boss.

After that night, table twenty-one became a cute "thing." Years later when Alonzo's closed, Peter called and asked if I wanted table twenty-one. Of course, I didn't hesitate to say yes, and it's been a permanent piece of furniture in my home ever since.

Then I went to the kitchen to check on the order

for my special customer. The chef was putting the finishing touches on it. He handed it to me, and I placed it on a tray and carried it to table twenty-one.

"Here's your food," I announced as I put the plate on the table in front of this handsome man.

He glanced around the restaurant. "Do you have a few minutes to sit down and chat while I eat?"

Surprised by his invitation, I thought, *Oh, my goodness. What have I gone and done?*

No doubt, my blushing became apparent, even in the soft lighting. Then I reminded myself, *This was what you wanted, Evelyn.*

I glanced over at Peter at the bar, which was nearby, close enough to be within earshot of him. I raised my eyebrows in a silent plea to let me linger at this table. Gratefully, he seemed to understand my request and nodded his approval, so I sat down across from my customer.

"I'm Bob, by the way. Bob Kormondy." He had yet to take a bite of his food and seemed more interested in me than it. He made me feel as if I was the only other person in the room . . . the only other person on this planet.

As I gazed into his eyes, I knew I was developing a strong attraction for this man, even though I didn't know his last name until now.

-2-

He's Back?

"Hi Bob Kormondy. I'm Evelyn. Evelyn Ashcroft."

His eyes bore into mine. "So, what do you do, Evelyn Ashcroft? Do you work here full time?"

"Actually, no. I only hostess at Alonzo's on the weekends because I really like working here. My daytime job is a bookkeeper and interior designer for my family's business."

He raised an eyebrow, signaling he was impressed. Then he finally took a bite of his manicotti.

"So, how about you, Bob Kormondy," I said, changing the subject. "I hear you work for NBC Sports. What do you do for them? What brought you to Jacksonville?"

"I'm a cameraman, and they send me to Jacksonville every year to work some of the Jaguars football games." His eyes and attention would only leave me to cut the food on his plate.

"That's right," I stated. "The Jaguars are playing tomorrow."

"Yep, and I'll be there to operate my camera." He gave a half-smile before taking another bite of his food.

"So what brings you to Alonzo's?" Whatever it was, I was thankful for it.

"Well," he started and then took a sip of water, "after checking into the hotel, I decided to go to a highly recommended Italian restaurant close by. I'd eaten here before and really enjoyed the food and atmosphere."

We continued to talk, mostly about his job, which seemed exciting. He told me about the different places around the world where NBC Sports had sent him so that he could cover different sporting events. The more he talked, the more confident and sexier he became. He definitely had my interest, and that marriage thought that had popped into my mind earlier, well, I could see that it could be a possibility after all. He was different from the other men I had met in that he spoke in a kind tone, and I liked that.

Bob finished his meal, but we still talked a few minutes more. I had to get back to work, so he walked with me to the front where he could pay his bill. Then I decided to make a bold move. While he was picking up his credit card and receipt, I handed him my name and phone number on a piece of paper, even though he hadn't asked for my number.

Despite my brazen actions, I couldn't hide my nervousness. However, I didn't want him to walk out of my life forever. "If you're back in Jacksonville and you and your crew want to know fun things to do while you're here, give me a call," I suggested.

He didn't say anything but instead, gave me a confident, sexy smile. I blushed from the embarrassment of being uncharacteristically forward. Then he took the piece of paper and left.

Through the door's glass panes, I watched as his back got smaller.

Rose walked over to stand next to me.

I sighed. "Gosh, I probably won't ever see him again." Even I could hear the disappointment in my voice. I turned and headed back to the cash register.

Rose stayed and kept her eyes fixed on the door. "Evelyn!" she exclaimed. "He's coming back up the walkway!"

I spun around to see what she was talking about, and there he was getting larger and larger as he got closer to the door. Overcome with excitement, I could hardly catch my breath. He walked back into the restaurant, and my heart raced at the sight of him standing in front of me.

"Evelyn, would you like to go dancing after you shift?"

Did he just ask me out on a date? My heart beat even faster! "I would enjoy going dancing after work," I replied while trying to remain calm, but inside, I was anything but.

His eyes twinkled. "Great! What time do you get off?"

Right now, I thought . . . I wished. "Eleven."

"Is there somewhere we can go?" he asked.

I thought for a moment as numerous places ran through my mind. "There's a place up the street called T-Birds," I suggested. I really didn't care where we went; anywhere would have been fine as long as I got to spend more time with him.

He smiled. "Okay then. I'll be back at eleven to go to T-Birds."

As he left, I turned around and saw the entire kitchen staff looking from the back of the restaurant and snickering. I didn't care, I was so ecstatic. For the rest of the night, almost all I could think about was my pending date.

As promised, Bob returned at eleven. He stepped into the lobby, and his smile made me feel as if he was truly happy to see me again.

"Ready?" he asked.

"Yep," I answered. "I'll drive my car, and you can follow me."

T-Birds was packed; it was Saturday night after all. Bob and I managed to navigate the crowd without getting separated. While trying to find a table, he shouted over the loud music, "Do you know anyone here?"

I shook my head. "No. I'm not a big party girl, so I rarely come here."

Surprisingly, however, Bob saw someone he knew. "Hey, there's a friend of mine," he yelled.

Crazy. Here I was a local girl and didn't know a soul in that whole crowded place, and along came Bob, an out-of-towner, and he did.

"He's working the Jacksonville Jaguars game to-morrow," he explained. "Would you like to meet him?"

I nodded instead of yelling back. Meeting people he called friends was a great way to learn more about him.

Bob's friend came over to table, and we all talk-ed for a while. I liked him; he seemed like a good per-son, which told me a lot about Bob. We talked about Jacksonville, and somehow during our conversation, the topic of my five sisters came up.

Then his friend pulled out two tickets for the next day's game and held them in front of me. "Evelyn, would you like these two tickets?" he asked. "You can take one of your sisters with you."

I glanced over at Bob. He nodded his head in encouragement.

"Absolutely!" I exclaimed. "I would love to have them. Thank you!"

A few minutes later, his friend went home, leav-ing Bob and me alone again, well, alone in a club full of people. We had so much fun that night. We danced and talked and danced and talked and got to know each other better. Periodically, I would catch him gaz-ing at me, and his big smile frequently told me that he liked being with me too.

Then he looked at his watch. "I gotta go," he stated, his voice sounding disappointed. "I gotta work tomorrow, and I need to be ready."

I understood, but I shared his disappointment. He walked me to my car. "I'm glad you're coming to the game tomorrow," he said. "If you'd like, we can meet up afterwards."

"Yes," I said as excitement bubbled up inside again. "I would like that."

He smiled. "Great!" Then he paused as he stared deeply into my eyes. "Evelyn, would you be okay if I gave you a kiss on the cheek?"

My heart fluttered inside as I tried to remain calm, cool, and collected on the outside. His question wasn't only about the kiss (although that was exciting enough!), but it meant that he respected me. It made me believe I meant something to him.

"Yes," I answered.

I turned my cheek toward him. He leaned over and smiled. He put his hand on the small of my back and pulled me toward him before giving me a soft, gentle kiss on the cheek.

Wow! That was far sexier than anything else he could have done!

As I drove through the parking lot, I glanced in my rearview mirror and saw him still standing where I had left him. Oddly, I felt protected, that he was watching after me to make sure I was safe.

Then he called me after I got home to make sure I made it home okay. My heart fluttered.

He added, "I'm looking forward to seeing you tomorrow."

"Me too," I agreed. "How do I find you after the game?"

"Ask one of the security guards where the NBC compound is. I'll meet you there."

He couldn't see me nodding, and thankfully, he couldn't hear me thinking, *Bob Kormondy, I'll find you. I don't care where you are; I'll find you!*

Lying in bed that night, all I could do was reflect on all that had transpired over the last several hours. What a night! All in all, by the end of it, I knew I wanted to spend more time with Bob Kormondy.

-3-

A Long Time Coming

The next day when I arrived at the football stadium with my sister Ginger, we discovered we had wonderful tickets on the fifty-yard line about four rows up. Premium seats located close to where the game would be played!

I glanced around to find Bob as soon as we got settled. "I wonder where Bob is," I mumbled, speaking my thoughts out loud.

"Evie, did he give you any clue as to where he might be assigned to film the game?" Ginger asked. "This is a big stadium."

"No," I answered ruefully.

This was a big stadium, so I should have asked, but I didn't. At the time, my mind wasn't *on* the game but on meeting him *after* the game.

But now, I wanted to see him in action doing his job. Actually, I just wanted to see him, even if it was from afar. My eyes darted all around, scouring the field and sidelines until they fell on a familiar person holding a camera!

"There he is!" I exclaimed and pointed to Bob. "He's the one on the camera lift on the field."

My sister's eyes followed mine. "Oh yes, I see him." She laughed. "Do you have a Bob radar?"

"I think I do," I answered with a big grin. Just seeing him there excited me as well as gave me comfort.

As we watched the game, I felt a light tap on the back of my shoulder. I turned around to see the gentleman sitting behind us looking directly at me. Using his thumb to point behind him, he said, "There's a lady sitting a couple of rows up who wants me to get your attention."

I looked to where he was pointing and recognized my sister Shirley and her husband, who was also named Bob. I ran up to talk to them.

"What are you doing here, Evie?" she asked. "And how did you get better seats than us?"

I turned my head to make sure that Bob was still where I had last seen him, and he was. "See that cameraman on the field?" I tilted my head in Bob's direction.

Shirley stretched her neck to look past me to explore the field. "Oh yeah, I see him," she answered.

"His friend gave the tickets to me. But the guy on the field, his name's Bob, and I'm going to marry him." My tone was resolved and determined and matter-of-fact.

Both she and my brother-in-law started laughing.

"Sure, you are," Shirley jeered.

"No," I insisted. "He's the one."

Shirley reduced her teasing to a smile, but her eyes still reflected skepticism.

They'll see, I thought. Deep down, there wasn't any question as to whether I would marry Bob Kormondy, so their responses of doubt didn't shake my confidence one bit.

Toward the end of the fourth quarter, anticipation built at the thought of being with Bob again, and I could hardly wait. I tried hard to act nonchalant around my sister, but it was challenging.

Finally, the game was over. I almost jumped out of my seat so that I could go and meet him. "We need to find a security guard to ask them where the compound is," I told my sister.

Asking a security guard was the easy part. He didn't hesitate to lead us to the entrance of the compound.

The challenging part was after he left. The guard who stood in front of the compound wouldn't let us in because we didn't have the required credentials.

Glancing around, I saw someone approaching the gate. He looked to have the credentials we needed. "Excuse me," I started, "We're looking for Bob Kormondy. He asked us to meet him here."

He studied us. After a couple of moments, he must have decided that we weren't a threat, so he said, "Sure, follow me." We did, and he brought us into the compound. "Wait here," he told us.

Within a few moments, I spotted Bob's friend, who I had met the previous night at T-Birds. He walked over to us.

"Waiting for Bob?" he asked.

I nodded, perhaps a bit too enthusiastically. "Yes. He said to come here and meet him."

"Okay. He's still on the field, but he should be here soon. I'll let him know you're here."

A few minutes later, Bob appeared. We greeted each other with a hug, and I introduced him to my sister. He took us further into the compound, introducing us to his coworkers and network colleagues along the way. He then gave us a tour and showed us the inside of the TV trucks and how the telecasts were put together and edited. He spoke with knowledge, confidence, and passion. It was incredibly interesting and exciting to learn about his work as well as see what his camera looked like up close.

I noticed earlier that when Bob was on the field working, he appeared extremely focused, his camera fixed on the ball. But now when he wasn't working, he was entirely focused on me, just like last night in the restaurant and then at T-Birds. It was a wonderful feeling.

That November 1995 football game started Bob and me on a lifetime adventure together. We spoke to each other every day on the phone because he lived in Tallahassee or was in some other city covering a sporting event. The more we got to know each other, the more I realized we shared the same values and had the same fundamental perspective—work hard and experience life to the fullest.

We also discovered that our lifestyles fit together perfectly. Sure, he traveled a lot, but I was fine with that. Sometimes, he would ask me to travel with him.

Our meeting was undoubtedly God-ordained because I learned that Bob had been just as attracted to me as I had been to him when we first met. Neither of us was expecting to meet the love of our life that night, but that was exactly what happened. In fact, Bob later told me, "When I entered the restaurant that evening, I had manicotti on my mind. However, as soon as I met you, the menu got a lot more memorable."

After a couple of years of dating, Bob brought his three school-age daughters into my life, and I was overjoyed. I believed that being a mom would never happen to me because eleven years prior to then, when I was only twenty-seven, I was diagnosed with cancer and had to undergo a hysterectomy. Fortunately, the doctors were able to remove all of the cancer from me, but it left me barren at such a young age. It truly saddened me because I wanted children so much. So you can only imagine how his daughters filled a void and were such an answer to prayer.

Bob and I weren't in a hurry to get married. We wanted to take the time to get to know each other and fall deeply in love so that when we became husband and wife, we would spend forever together. It was also important to him that I get to know his daughters and vice-versa and for them to be comfortable with me and love me.

God made that happen. He showed me that I didn't need to be fertile to be a mom. As I got to know Bob's daughters more, a motherly connection to them grew and flourished. Embracing that blessed role of mother started to naturally occur. One day, they would be my daughters, and I would be a "bonus mom" to them. And through a powerful grace, their mom shared them with me.

It was all a process, and truthfully, I wasn't in a rush anyways. I had been single for a very long time and consequently, was independent. I had changed jobs since meeting Bob; actually, I had changed careers. My father's shop had closed, and I went back to school to become a neuromuscular therapist and then started working for my sister Shirley's clinic.

On the night of March 8, 2001, I had just prepared Bob's favorite dinner in the kitchen of my apartment. Cooking for him had become part of our routine when he came to town to visit me, so there was nothing out of the ordinary that would clue me in that in a few moments, my life would change forever.

Before I could take my first bite, he stood up un-expectedly and walked over to me. He bent down and kissed me before taking my hand in his. "Evie, I love you very much. I want to spend the rest of my life with you. Will you marry me?"

Of course, I said yes! I was so happy!

He grinned from ear to ear. "I'm sorry I don't have a ring to give you now, but I figured you could pick it out. How about we go shopping tomorrow for a beauti-ful ring for that beautiful finger of yours?"

I thought, *I'll go to the moon with you, Bob Kormondy.* "Absolutely!" I answered.

We then kissed to seal the deal.

The next day, Bob took me to a jewelry store. "Pick out what you'd like, Evie."

I didn't know what he wanted to spend, so I chose two rings but in two completely different price ranges. Honestly, I didn't really care which ring I had. It was more about marrying him and being his wife.

After putting the least expensive ring on my finger, I held out my hand to Bob for him to evaluate. I did the same with the most expensive ring. After a few sec-onds, he decided upon what I called the "21-gun salute" because it had twenty-one diamonds and was absolutely gorgeous!

And I was ecstatic! "How did you know I wanted that one?" I asked.

"Because your eyes lit up when you put it on, sweetheart." He shrugged. "Hey, I was paying attention."

We left the jewelry store with that beautiful ring on my finger and drove to my parents' house. I gave them the news about our engagement and held my hand out for them to admire my new ring. They were thrilled because they had come to love Bob as a son and knew how happy he made me. Mom hugged him, and Dad shook his hand with a big smile.

Next stop . . . my sister's Shirley's clinic. We worked together every day, so we would often talk and confide in each other. She knew how much I loved Bob and how long I had been waiting to find my perfect man and someday marry him.

Shirley was standing at the receptionist desk when we walked in. I didn't say anything, just held my left hand in front of her. No way could she miss that ring.

She paused a moment. Then it was like a lightbulb went off. She started screaming in excitement and ran over to hug me and then Bob. All the therapists, who were my colleagues, came out of their rooms to find out what all the commotion was about.

Shirley exclaimed, "Bob and Evie just got engaged! They're getting married!"

The commotion then escalated as the therapists joined in and started squealing too.

That night, Bob had to leave for another assignment. Once he got settled into his hotel room in another city, he called me. "Evie, how can we be in two different states after just getting engaged? We should be together, celebrating."

I agreed, but we would be together soon enough. After all, we had been together for over five years thus far.

There was so much to do to plan a wedding, something I had done in my head for as long as I've known Bob Kormondy. Now that we were engaged, we needed to set the date so that I could get busy getting that stuff out of my head and actually putting together my dream wedding.

The next time Bob was in town, we set our wedding date for January 12, 2002.

– 4 –

"I Do"

Shopping for my wedding dress with my mother will always remain with me as a special memory. We found a stunning white chiffon gown with a beautiful veil. When I tried it on at the store and saw myself in the mirror, I felt like a princess.

Then we took Bob's daughters shopping for their bridesmaids' dresses and had so much fun with them. They were so thrilled to be in the ceremony. The twins, Kristy and Michelle, were twelve, and Charlene was only nine. She was so tiny, but she wanted her dress to match her sisters' dresses. We ended up buying her the smallest-size bridesmaid dress available and still had it cut down more. We also picked out a dress for my five-year-old great niece, Sabrina, who would be my flower girl.

Before we knew it, our wedding day had arrived. Bob and I had bought a home in anticipation of our marriage, and our three girls had spent the night with me there. When we woke up, we were all excited. We ate breakfast, played the song "Going to the Chapel," and had my friend, a professional hairdresser, come over to do our hair and put makeup on us. We were all ready except for putting on our dresses, which we planned to do at the church.

Bob was at the hotel with his brother and friends. He called several times. During one of his calls, he said, "Sweetheart, you're not here at the chapel. Where are you?"

"Bob, I'm at the house with the girls. Honey, it's only 3:00. The wedding's not until six."

"Uhm, Evie, it's 5:40," he informed me.

What? My heart skipped a few beats. I looked at my watch, and its hands weren't moving. *Oh my goodness! My watch stopped!* I never bothered to look at the clocks scattered around the house.

I had thought the limo driver had arrived early, so I told him to sit on the couch to wait for us, even gave him something to drink. He never mentioned anything about the time.

The girls and I jumped into the limo laughing hard. But I was a little panicked inside; I didn't want the girls to know. To this day, Bob still teases me about my being late to my own wedding, and we laugh about it.

When we finally arrived at the church, we rushed inside and put our dresses on. The photographer took a few pictures with my mom and dad and the girls. Then I was off to meet my man.

My dad took my arm, and I gazed into his eyes. He asked, "Are you ready, little girl?"

"Yes, Daddy, I am."

He led me down the aisle, and at the other end stood my prince, who was very soon to be my husband. My eyes never left him the whole way.

By the time we got married, we had dated for over six years. I was forty-two years old on our wedding day, and it was my first and still is my only marriage. The ceremony turned out to be absolutely beautiful with about 150 friends and family members in attendance. Dr. Garrett married us in my church of thirty-five years, and it was the last wedding he officiated before retiring.

All the girls did such a good job; I was so proud of them. They were now my family and would be for the rest of my life. I had to be the luckiest woman in the entire world.

After the ceremony, a horse-drawn carriage pulled in front of the church to take us to the reception. January can get pretty cold in Florida, and the evening temperatures were dropping. I only had a white floor-length cape to wear over my dress. But I didn't care. I was now married to the most wonderful man in the world!

We climbed up into the carriage. The girls watched with smiles. When they turned to leave and get into the car with my mom and dad, I yelled, "Oh no. You girls are up here in the carriage with us."

They spun around, their eyes flying wide open in surprise. They ran over to the carriage and climbed into the seat across from us. Bob smiled at me so tenderly in that moment.

As the horse plodded down Baymeadows Road, the passing cars honked their horns. The girls waved and waved and had so much fun.

The reception was held in a large ballroom at the Embassy Suites. We offered a sit-down dinner to the guests. Everyone danced and seemed to enjoy themselves, including our daughters and my niece Sabrina. The night turned out to be a big hit for all.

The next day, Bob and I left for our honeymoon in Cancun, Mexico. It was a dream wedding, a dream reception, and a dream honeymoon. Most important, though, it was the start of a dream life together as husband and wife!

−5−

Living the Dream

Bob's love for photography opened my eyes to the art of it. I discovered I was pretty good with a camera and fell in love shooting everything in sight, especially nature. So he started encouraging me and taught me how to develop my skills and talent. He was such a good, patient teacher, and I loved learning from him.

Then my love for sports and Bob transitioned me to specializing in sport shots. Before I knew it, I became a photographer for several professional sports teams in Jacksonville, shooting top sports professionals. Sometimes while Bob covered a game in real time with his camera, I shot pictures of the game with my camera.

In July 2010, Bob was working the annual American Century Celebrity Golf Championship in Lake Tahoe, and I was there for the first time as a photographer for a magazine. Charles Barkley, the professional basketball player, was one of the participants. Everyone seemed to want a picture with him, including all the professional photographers from different media outlets all over the world. They kept clamoring out his name, wanting to shoot photos of him on the golf course.

However, I'm not a yeller. I had managed to get close enough to him, though. Then during a rare quiet moment, I softly asked, "Mr. Barkley, may I have a photo please?"

All of a sudden, Mr. Barkley stopped. "Hey, everybody, be quiet." He then looked around. "Who just asked, 'May I have a photo please?'"

I raised my hand. "That was me, Mr. Barkley."

A big grin spread across his face. "Little Voice, Little Voice, come over here."

Now, nervousness spread across my whole being, but I did what he told me to do and walked over to him.

"Stand right here," he instructed.

Then he shouted out the names of his friends, who were also playing in the tournament, to join him in a photo shoot. They all gathered in a group and posed in a picture for me. He wouldn't let the other photographers shoot this picture, letting them know that it was an exclusive just for me.

Every time he saw me after that event, he would say, "Little Voice, Little Voice." It always put a smile on my face and gave me confidence as a first-time photographer on the golf course.

While I grew in my career, Bob excelled in his as a network camera operator for NBC Sports, a job he cherished and one that has awarded him six Emmys. Both his job and the Emmys were no small feat but the fruit of his lifelong hard work. To him, though, it wasn't work; it was being given the opportunity to get up close and personal with his passion. It enabled him to cover major sports events all around the world, such as the Olympics, Ryder Cups, US Opens, The Masters, the British Open tournaments, and Super Bowls.

Not only did our careers complement each other, but our activities during our time off did as well. Bob and I either participated in sports together or I cheered him on in a support capacity whenever I could. Sometimes, though, other commitments got in my way, and I would have to tend to them instead. We were both good with that, giving each other some independence.

I also recognized that Bob needed to stay active on his days off with or without me. Whereas some people relaxed when not at work, he unwound from the stress by engaging in some type of physical activity—golf, tennis, billiards, ice skating, mountain biking, paddle boarding, archery, surfing, and windsurfing. He even tested brand-new windsurf boards for windsurfing magazines.

Of course, he was always better than me in almost every sport, although there was a time when I had one up on him with my golf short game. I was quite proud of myself since Bob was quite the golfer. He just shrugged it off and retorted, "Well, Evie, seems like Putt Putt's worked really well for you." We both enjoyed a good laugh.

Bob never found life boring, and neither did I. Even when he was away, which was quite often due to his job, we both kept busy. Still, I missed him so much during those times.

But in a way, his absences were also a good thing. The time alone allowed me to get some projects out of the way. He would then come home for a short time, rest and recoup, and then we would be right back at it, active with sports and friends. After about a week or so, he would have to go back on the road again.

And as often as possible, I traveled with him. Traveling together brought us closer, and it also blessed us with friends all over the country as well as in England, Ireland, Italy, Greece, Scotland, and Australia.

We truly enjoyed our highly active lifestyle, but on a foundational level, we truly enjoyed each other, to be in each other's presence. We've never stopped dating and exploring each other, even after our nuptials. We've been each other's best friend, and together, we've grown closer to God.

Bob and I had it all. Great family, great marriage, great careers, and we had both survived cancer—me at the age of twenty-seven, and Bob in 2009 after a three-year battle with vocal cord cancer. We believed we had faced and conquered the worst of it. Life was good; life was fun, and we were having a blast doing it.

And then in a blink of an eye, it flipped upside down.

I never saw it coming!

–6–

What's Wrong?

November 02, 2011—the day started like any other day for Bob and me—coffee and homemade scones. He would eat every bite on his plate with such enthusiasm. I couldn't help but wonder if it was because he was on the road so much and finally had a home-cooked meal or if I was a great cook or both. Not that it mattered. He simply enjoyed the food I cooked for him, and that made me happy. In the meantime, I had him home with me.

Soon after breakfast, he left to go windsurfing, and I had to stay behind because I had a busy day in front of me. Then around 5:00 p.m., I started preparing dinner. The marinating steaks would be ready to cook in about thirty minutes, and I was just about finished making our salads. Bob called and said he would be home in about fifteen minutes. Perfect. By the time he arrived and got cleaned up, dinner would be ready.

The front door opened and closed, signaling Bob was home. "I'm in the kitchen," I yelled over my shoulder while washing the last of the dirty dishes.

I turned to greet him but froze as soon as I saw the right side of his neck. It was tremendously swollen.

"What happened to your neck?" I asked, both concerned and confused. "Did something bite you?" The more I studied how enlarged it was, the more worried I became. "Should we go to the emergency room?"

"Nah," he shrugged. "I don't think anything bit me. I think I might have pulled a muscle in it though."

I accepted his answer without further questions. However, while he was in the shower, my concern grew. The swelling brought back to memory the vocal cord cancer he had from 2006 to 2009. During that time, the doctors did two successful scrapings on him that removed the cancer. At the end, he was given a clean bill of health, and that was two years ago. We had hardly thought about it since everything had gone so well, but now, I couldn't dismiss it.

We talked about his neck over dinner. He told me how it started hurting while he was windsurfing, so it only made sense that he must have injured himself at that time. The possibility of him being bitten by something was still on the table for me.

By the end of dinner, I felt much better about his condition. Still, I wanted to be cautious. We were leaving in a few days to go to Australia for two weeks. Bob had to work the Presidents Cup Golf Tournament there, and then we would extend our stay and have a vacation. It would be a relief to figure out what was wrong with his neck before we left so that we could enjoy ourselves.

"I think it would be a good idea if you got it checked out by Dr. Tucker before we go to Australia," I suggested.

"Okay," he agreed. "We can call him first thing in the morning."

Dr. Clark Tucker had been Bob's ear, nose, and throat doctor for the three years he had vocal cord cancer.

First thing the next day, on November 3, as soon as Dr Tucker's office opened, I was on the phone with his receptionist. I explained the situation and that we were going out of the country in a few days. We were then told to come in at 11:30 that morning.

When Dr. Tucker entered the examination room, we expected a smile and warm welcome. Instead, his eyes remained fixed on Bob's neck, and no smile appeared on his face. Both his nurse and Amy, his assistant, had concerned expressions with furrowed brows and slightly opened mouths. None of them reassured us that this was a minor problem.

The unknown started to create apprehension, and my heart beat a little faster. I squeezed Bob's hand in encouragement even though it was something I wished I had myself.

Dr. Tucker began his examination. I watched his every move and strained to listened to every one of his questions and Bob's answers to them.

"This doesn't have anything to do with vocal cord cancer," he announced.

Whew! My body relaxed. Relief! But it was short-lived.

"I do feel something dramatic's going on," he proclaimed. "I'd like to take aspirations of several sections of Bob's neck and send them for biopsy."

My eyes popped open in surprise. Biopsies? Aspirations? Confusion. Disbelief.

"But we're leaving for Australia in a few days, and we'll be gone for two weeks," Bob argued.

"Good thing I have a new machine then. I can do the aspirations right here right now. You're the first to use it," Dr. Tucker explained, trying to lighten the cloud of heaviness that had enveloped us. He then left the room and us with our thoughts.

Even at his assertion that something dramatic was going on and his suggestion of doing aspirations and biopsies, Dr. Tucker seemed more optimistic than how he looked when he first saw Bob's neck. He had since had a chance to examine it, so surely, it was an infection or something else that was very treatable. No reason to panic.

A few minutes later, Dr. Tucker returned and told us that we needed to change rooms. So I grabbed our belongings, and we followed him down the hall. He pointed to a chair. "Sit there, Bob. It leans back, so make yourself comfortable and lie back for me."

The nurse came in pushing a machine on wheels and parked it next to Bob. Dr. Tucker applied a local anesthetic onto his neck before doing the aspirations from the swollen lymph nodes. The third area was a rock-solid mass, so it took a lot of effort to penetrate it and extract enough of a sample for a biopsy. Thankfully, the anesthetic must have worked because Bob didn't appear to be in any pain.

In just a few minutes, the procedure was over. Dr. Tucker said, "Go ahead, and have fun in Australia, but come back to see me as soon as you return. I'll have the results by then, and we can talk at that time."

I asked, "Dr. Tucker, do you have any idea what could be causing the swelling?" I had more questions now than I did before.

He shook his head. "Can't say."

His demeanor didn't reveal any more than his two-word answer. We all knew there was something abnormal going on with Bob's neck, and infections are not normal. In fact, anything that is contrary to perfect health should be considered abnormal.

We left his office and decided to go have lunch somewhere, really not giving Bob's visit with Dr. Tucker anymore thought. In our minds, the swelling would go down while we were in Australia, and we would have a good time. Then when we returned, Dr. Tucker would tell us it was some kind of infection and prescribe some kind of medicine to treat it if it was still a problem.

Afterwards, Bob's neck would heal, and we would go on with our everyday lives.

−7−

Australia, Here We Come!

Five days later, on November 8, 2011, we boarded a plane to Australia. I had never been there, so I was so thrilled, knowing we would have an amazing trip. The flight, however, was so very long—twenty hours and seven minutes with layovers. By the time we arrived, I was glad I wouldn't have to board a plane for another two weeks.

The swelling in Bob's neck had not diminished any, but he nevertheless functioned fine during the Presidents Cup Golf Tournament. However, he started noticing some restriction in turning his head to the left or right but not enough for concern. If anything, the inability to fully turn his head increased our belief that it was an injured neck muscle. So we set out to have fun and focus solely on what we were doing at the time. Anything beyond that was out of sight, out of mind.

After the tournament, we went forth with our vacation full throttle and had the time of our lives! We visited Torquay, a wonderful little beach town. The people were as nice as they could be. And of course, what would a vacation be if sports weren't involved? So Bob paddle boarded and surfed as well as windsurfed with some new Australian friends. In fact, we met so many people while there, and to this day, we still have dear friends in Australia.

We also attended our one and only cricket match and sat on the bench with the team. Then we played golf on another day. During one of our games, several kangaroos came onto the course and hopped all around.

At one point while I was talking with Bob, I heard what sounded like thunder coming up behind me. I turned around and saw a kangaroo hopping toward us. He scared me so much that I ran up into Bob's arms, yelling, "Oh my goodness! Oh my goodness!"

Bob just laughed and put his arms around me protectively. "He's okay," he assured me. "He's just passing by us."

He was right. The kangaroo hopped to the closest tree to eat some leaves. When he stood on his hindlegs, he looked to be at least seven feet tall, which surprised me. These kangaroos were so much fun, and we enjoyed some good laughs at their fearlessness. One of them carried a baby in her pouch.

Sightseeing was a must. We fed some parrots and were delighted to come across koala bears in the wild. They were so adorable that I wanted to hold them. So Bob took me to find a place that had koalas to hold. We learned that visitors weren't allowed to hold koalas because they don't have rib cages and could easily be injured. So we resorted to enjoying looking at their cute little faces from a distance.

In the midst of all our fun, it wasn't hard to see that Bob's neck continued to swell even more. We continued to be encouraged that everything was okay, and once we got back home, it would go away once treated.

However, toward the end of our trip, he couldn't turn his neck very well, but my Bob just kept on having fun anyway. He was pretty amazing, refusing to let it keep him from enjoying every moment we were there together.

Our wonderful Australian adventure turned out to be a mini-honeymoon. I am truly blessed to have such an amazing husband, one who has shown me so many adventures throughout our lives together.

And Australia, well, that was one we would remember for the rest of our lives.

– 8 –

The Diagnosis

We were back in the States on November 23 and were greeted with a voicemail from Dr. Tucker. "Come to my office as soon as you get back from Australia. No appointment's necessary. Just come."

I became more than concerned by his message. As a knee-jerk reaction, I glanced at the clock to see if Dr. Tucker's office was still open. Then I reminded myself that it was after-hours, so I would need to call in the morning. Fortunately, the next day was Thursday, a weekday, so we should be able to go and see him then.

Not so fast. Turned out, Dr. Tucker wouldn't be in his office until Monday. We would have to wait almost five days to find out why he needed Bob to see him as soon as we returned.

During that time, Bob and I prayed; it was all we could do. We knew that whatever it was, God would help us through it

First thing Monday morning, however, we were sitting in Dr. Tucker's waiting room. His staff didn't come across as open and friendly as they had been in the past; they were just quieter than what we were used to. Maybe we were just scared, but it seemed as if everyone was walking on eggshells and treating us like, "Oh my gosh! The Kormondys are here."

A nurse called Bob's name a few minutes later, and we followed her down the hall and into Dr. Tucker's office, which was also something we weren't used to. Usually, we would be taken to an exam room. Bob and I looked at each other, his confused expression mirroring my own.

As we entered, my eyes fell upon the large wooden desk. We sat down in the two black chairs in front of it. I felt so small in comparison. I grabbed Bob's hand and squeezed it, and I wouldn't let it go.

Then Dr. Tucker walked in. He was serious during our previous visit, but now, he was intense. In fact, the last time I had seen him with such an ominous expression was when Bob had gotten diagnosed with vocal cord cancer.

"Bob," he started, staring into my husband's

eyes, "I got your test results back." He briefly searched Bob's face. "It's neck and throat cancer," he pronounced.

Someone sucked the air out of the room. *What? I must not have heard you correctly. Bob's healthy. No way could he have cancer . . . again!* I fought the urge to not throw up right then and there.

I looked at Bob, waiting for him to do or say something to dispute those words, to speak what I was thinking. Instead, he sat there silent, stunned, his eyes fixed on Dr. Tucker and his mouth slightly ajar. I could tell he was trying to make sense out of those three words, the same ones that didn't make sense to me either.

"But we got rid of his cancer two years ago!" I argued what I thought was the obvious.

Dr. Tucker glanced at me without responding. Then he placed his eyes back onto my husband. "Bob?" he asked.

It appeared as if Dr. Tucker's one-word question broke Bob out of his stupor. He stared at me, and I stared at him, both of us with tears in our eyes. It was all very emotional with too many unanswered questions.

Finally, I found my voice and spoke, not taking my eyes off of Bob. "Can we redo the biopsies? Maybe they're wrong."

Dr. Tucker stared at me. He pursed his lips and shook his head.

"Okay, then who's the very best surgeon, and where's he located?" We had to hit this head-on by getting him the best care as soon as possible. We were going to do our part, no matter what it was.

Dr. Tucker let out a deep breath and shrugged. "Dr. Simpson. The good news is that he's here in Jacksonville. The bad news is that you can't get an appointment with him. He has a wait-list of about a month, and there's no way Bob can wait that long."

I tried to process this news, but rational thinking had been left behind with the words "it's neck and throat cancer." Bob looked so lost, as if the determination and resolve a few moments earlier seemed to have completely disappeared, and hope had been yanked out of him.

Immediately, my heart slowed down, and a peace came over me. At first, I didn't understand why, but then it hit me. Church had always been a big part of my life. My parents and I were some of the founding members of our church, and we've watched it grow in every way over the years. I've taught vacation Bible school for so long, I can't remember when I started. God has been front and center in my life, and after Bob and I married, He became front and center in our lives together.

As a child of God, we have power through the name of Jesus. We sometimes don't realize that power until we really need it. In that instance sitting in front of Dr. Tucker, I needed it, and it was there!

I leaned forward in my chair with the excitement that comes from an epiphany that's dropped into your spirit when you realize you just experienced a miracle. "Dr. Tucker, did you say Dr. Simpson? Is that Dr. Lee Simpson?"

Dr. Tucker's eyebrows furrowed a little in confusion as his head tilted slightly to the side. "Yes."

My heart fluttered in joy as I sat back in my chair full of confidence. I'll never forget that moment. What had been a normal part of my life was now going to save my husband's life.

Bob and Dr. Tucker stared at me perplexed.

With a huge grin on my face, I stated, "Dr. Tucker, please call Dr. Simpson immediately and tell him that Evelyn Ashcroft is asking him to see her husband for throat cancer."

"Evelyn, that's not possible," Dr. Tucker repeated.

"Please, Dr. Tucker. Please call."

He shrugged but picked up the phone and dialed. I could only hear his side of the conversation, but I knew what the outcome would be, nevertheless.

Dr. Tucker laid the receiver in its cradle, shrugged, and glanced at me before looking at Bob. "I don't understand. You have a 7:00 a.m. appointment in three days."

But I understood. By the grace of God, I had worked as a receptionist for Dr. Simpson thirty-two years ago. Of all people to work for . . . God knew what laid ahead for me, that my husband, the person I loved more than anything in the world, would need the best surgeon in the world thirty-two years later, and so He put me with that surgeon. It was a connection that I would need to reestablish. I knew what kind of physician and person Dr. Simpson was behind the scenes. He had always treated his staff like family, and he never forgot anyone.

We now had hope, but it didn't take away the seriousness of Bob's diagnosis. That night, I don't think either of us slept. We held each other and cried a lot. We even questioned the test results. Maybe they were wrong. We thanked God for His mercy and goodness, for pointing out to me my connection with Dr. Simpson.

Lying in the dark, I considered the alternative. What would it have been like to go home without knowing that Bob would be in the hands of the best surgeon?

God had opened a door for us. We would hold on tight to that door for today and take tomorrow as it came. However, the miracle of today gave us the confidence to move into tomorrow.

– 9 –

Four Months to Live

Before seeing Dr. Simpson, Bob had to undergo a series of tests so that he would know for sure what he was contending with. So we stayed busy with appointments for bloodwork, an EKG, Pet Scan, MRI, and other invasive tests that would wear anyone out. We would then go home and get on our knees and pray for a miracle.

Then on November 29, three days after seeing Dr. Tucker, we entered the waiting room of Dr. Simpson's office and signed in at the large desk to the right of the door. Fortunately, it was early, so the room was empty. From the size of it, though, and from the wait list that Dr. Tucker told us Dr. Simpson had, I could only imagine what it looked like when it was full.

A few moments later, the receptionist called Bob's name. He walked over to her and announced who he was. She handed him a clipboard with a stack of forms on it. "Please fill these out, Mr. Kormondy. In the meantime, if you could give me your insurance card and driver's license, I'll make a copy of them and get them back to you."

I watched Bob lumber back to his seat. Even though I knew the clock was moving at a normal pace, I could still physically feel the tick tock, tick tock of each second. Even though we were both very much in shock as to why we were there, I figured I would probably be able to focus more on completing the forms. So I took the clipboard from him and began filling them out.

Bob sat next to me, his facial muscles tense. He whispered the answers as we went through the questions. Then I would hand him the forms he needed to sign. He would put his signature on them without even looking at what they were.

It was a lot to process, and now he was having to put his life in the hands of a stranger. He had never met Dr. Simpson, so he didn't share the same confidence level as me. Last night, I tried to assure him that he was a brilliant surgeon and reminded him of the accolades that Dr. Tucker had bestowed upon him and his skills. I think Bob was coming around, but he would know soon enough when he talked to him.

As soon as we completed all of the paperwork, I gave them to the receptionist, and she led us down the hallway to an examination room. No sooner did we get settled than Dr. Simpson came in. He shook Bob's hand. For a moment, Bob relaxed a bit. Although I expected this, I was nevertheless relieved that Bob seemed more comfortable.

Dr. Simpson turned and smiled at me. He then warmly shook my hand. "Good to see you, Evelyn."

Two other doctors joined us in the small exam room. Dr. Simpson pointed to them one by one. "Bob, this is Dr. Jack Martin. He'll be your radiation oncologist. And this is Dr. Ed Brock, your medical oncologist."

We all nodded to each other.

Dr. Simpson then started the examination. Unlike Dr. Tucker prior to the aspirations, no local anesthetic was applied. So when he touched or pushed certain areas, Bob would grimace as his body tensed up or recoiled from the pain. It was as if I could feel it with him.

Then the other two doctors took turns examining Bob as well. Each held serious and concerned expressions. Nausea stirred inside me, and I willed myself to stay calm for Bob.

More and more doctors—internists and interns—came in. As the room filled, I was pushed farther and farther back until I was against the wall. Apparently, Bob's case was quite unusual. Since Dr. Simpson's office was part of Mercy teaching hospital, they were all interested. They studied his neck, and some touched it and gazed at it with amazement as if they had never seen something like that before. They murmured between themselves in words I couldn't comprehend. What was comprehensible, though, was their deep apprehension.

I wanted to stand next to Bob and hold his hand, but I felt as if I was looking at him through a constantly narrowing tunnel. We both started crying as the exam and conversation between the three main doctors continued.

When Dr. Simpson started asking him questions, a hush fell over the room. Bob didn't answer; instead, he sat there in silence. I think he was too stunned to say anything, so I yelled out the answer for him from the back of the room.

Dr. Simpson leaned closer to Bob. "I've reviewed all of your test results, Bob. You have neck and throat cancer with multiple masses of cancer growths, starting from the back of your tonsils and going down the right side of your neck and under your shoulder." He paused, allowing his explanation to sink in. "You're going to need a radical neck dissection."

A *what*?

Bob I and now stared at each other. He looked just as confused as I felt. I didn't know what this meant in context to Bob's life, but it all sounded very bad.

Dr. Simpson continued. "We're going to remove your tonsils, lymph nodes, salivary glands, neck muscles on the right side, shoulder muscles across the top of your right shoulder, and we're going to remove the cancer."

Oh, dear God! That was a mouthful of things they were going to remove. Now I understood why they called it "radical dissection." It sounded as if they were dissecting everything in and around his neck! Would he have anything left?

But Dr. Simpson wasn't done. "You're then going to need massive radiation and chemotherapy."

He studied Bob's motionless face. "Bob, this dissection is the best treatment, and it'll be a successful treatment. You'll still be able to enjoy the life you were accustomed to. You'll be able to lead normal lives."

Would we? How? This didn't make sense. Bob led a physical life. When he wasn't operating a camera for his job, he was windsurfing in thirty-five-mile-per-hour winds during his time off.

"But . . ." Dr. Simpson interrupted my string of internal questions.

Oh, how I hate the word "but."

"Your lives will have a new normal with restrictions," he added.

What did that mean? Was he trying to just calm us down, let us down easy? My mind was bursting with more questions.

Bob remained speechless, so I continued to talk for him. "Dr. Simpson, of course, we're shocked, but are you sure he needs to have all that done? What if we don't want to do all of that?"

Dr. Simpson's eyes bore into Bob's. "Evelyn, there are a number of things we must do immediately, or Bob has only four months to live."

Now I felt as if someone just hit me across the chest with a sledgehammer. I hadn't even processed that the love of my life had cancer, and now we're being told he had only four months to live if we didn't comply with everything? These thoughts reverberated around my brain like an out-of-control ping pong ball.

After finally catching my breath, I said, "We need a moment alone." The doctors all nodded in understanding and left the room.

I walked over to Bob, and we held each other and cried. In between sobs, Bob asked, "Evelyn, did I hear him right? I mean, all I kept hearing was 'cut, cut, cut, cut, cut.' This is my neck; this is my life."

"Yes, Bob, you heard him right." I did *not* want to say those words.

"Did he really say I had only four months to live?" he whispered.

Again, I didn't want to give the answer, but I did. "Yes. We have to do whatever Dr. Simpson says. There's no way I'm going to lose you."

We prayed together for God to give us the strength to handle all that was going to come our way. After gathering ourselves, I opened the door for Dr. Simpson to come back into the room.

"Okay," I said. "We trust you. Whatever it takes."

He gave me a hug. "Evelyn, it'll be all right. I'm going to take good care of your husband."

I never doubted he would, but his words bolstered me anyway. Bob continued to look stunned, but his jaw became set, and he seemed ready for a fight that would get him back his life.

What else could we do? We had to go along with the plan. Otherwise, the consequences were not only unacceptable but beyond what I wanted to consider.

I found myself speaking my thoughts out loud. "Surgery first, and then we'll go back to the way we always were. We've been shaken out of our norm, and now we need to get into the now, one day at a time, and we can handle anything."

To my own ears, I sounded cliché, but I didn't care. Our focus would be what would help us most. Plus, Bob needed to hear my optimism and my belief in our tomorrow. But I was also centering myself back to today and reminding myself of our motto—tomorrow was what the calendar was for.

We held each other's hand as we walked to our car, both of us wet with tears and numb with news.

"Now, we'll focus on today," I announced. "And today, I have you, and you have me. For the moment, all is well. Moment by moment, we'll address each issue and fight through them until the calendar clears. Tomorrow, we'll share the news with our girls—that'll be the hardest. Then we'll tell the rest of the family and our pastor and our friends."

Bob listened without responding. Right now, he needed to be reassured and encouraged. In the car, I prayed for him and the upcoming surgery.

We did all we could for the day, and for now, that was enough.

−10−

Tick Tock, Tick Tock

Mornings were always a special time for Bob and me. They were one of the many small rituals that signaled the beginning of a new and wonderful day and a time when we talked and planned and laughed.

The morning of December 8 was different, though. For the first time in our daily routine together, we didn't start with coffee or breakfast due to the surgery. There was no planning and no laughing. We got dressed and made our conversation positive. The last six days had hovered over us, actually more like haunted us, so we were just glad it had finally arrived.

Granted, it would have been easier if the surgery happened the day after meeting with Dr. Simpson and before some of the numbness had subsided, but that wasn't possible. Bob had to undergo prepping and more testing for the surgery. Through it all, we held onto the blessing that we were able to get in to see Dr. Simpson and so quickly.

When we left the house at 5 a.m. to go to the hospital, it was still dark outside. It was also dark as to what laid ahead for us and how much time we had together.

I silently screamed, *Forever, forever, forever!* But what was forever? *Okay, then one hundred years,* I negotiated with myself. Fear and desperation started to flood through my body. *Evelyn,* I scolded, *you need to calm yourself for Bob's sake as well as your own.*

It felt all wrong to be heading west to the hospital instead of east to the beach, which was our natural habitat. I wanted to grab the steering wheel and turn the car around. Instead, I studied Bob's neck that was somewhat illuminated by the dashboard light. It didn't seem so bad now. He was as strong as ever, as kind as ever, and as wonderful as ever.

My eyes started tearing. I loved him so much. I didn't want anyone touching him, hurting him, or changing the life he loved, not one iota, no, not one!

We had done most of our talking last night, about how difficult it was for him to go into surgery knowing that he would never be the same afterward. The decision was out of our hands, though, because the only other option was not an option. This radical neck dis-section must be done for Bob to live.

Radical was such a harsh word, but so was the four-month death sentence that had been proclaimed over his life. Bob was very aware that he had to put himself in the hands of his doctor, who was still a stranger to him, and trust in his judgment and expertise.

We had prayed together and prayed with family and friends. In the end, it was God who would decide the outcome. And in that there was some peace.

The drive was mostly silent. We both were heavy in thought. I needed to hold it together and not allow myself to venture below the surface to places I didn't want to go until forced.

My stomach churned as the lights of the hospital neared. I dreaded what we were walking into while at the same time, I urgently wanted to get it over with. Bob seemed to be taking it well. He stood on his strength and faith in God, knowing that He would keep him safe and guide Dr. Simpson's hand to remove the cancer and start him on his recovery journey.

We checked into the surgical department right on time—5:45, but then much too soon, they called him back. I tried to be strong, but I wanted to keep holding his hand and keep him by my side.

Bob pulled away and hugged me. After he kissed me, he whispered in my ear, "I'll be all right." And then he was gone, and time completely stopped.

Lost, I stumbled back to the waiting room and fell into an empty seat. Tick tock, tick tock, tick tock. My mind filled with so many questions—What direction would our lives take? Would Bob survive the surgery? And if so, would he be told that it was so bad, he only had two weeks to live because they couldn't do anything for him? Would our prayers be answered as we're told the surgery was a success and then hope would surround us? Would he survive and have the chance to schedule the radiation and chemotherapy so that we could continue to fight for his life, my life, and our lives together?

My mind felt as if it had a wrecking ball swinging out of control. Bottom line: I couldn't see life without him.

I had asked family and friends to come later so that I could have Bob all to myself for those last few minutes. They started arriving, and from 8:00 on that morning, we all prayed. I felt enveloped by hundreds of thousands of prayers.

I've participated in many prayer circles like the one that surrounded us at that time. I know they were just as strong for the unknown person as they were for the family member. I then prayed for many blessings to rain down upon the person who shared the brilliant idea of prayer circles. As a result, my heart rate decreased from a million beats a minute to something much more normal, and I could think rationally again.

Tick tock, tick tock, tick tock. The surgery was supposed to take six hours, so why was it taking so long, more than eight hours that seemed like a hundred years. All kind of negative scenarios came creeping back into my head.

Finally, Dr. Simpson appeared around 5:30 that evening. Even though he looked exhausted, he was a welcome sight. He trudged over to me. "Bob did great, Evelyn. He's in recovery now. They'll come and get you soon to take you back to him. I'll be back here tomorrow and go over the details then."

I nodded in understanding and wanted to hug him in relief and from joy that Bob had made it through the surgery! He made it! We were moving forward! I waited eagerly to see my husband.

Turning around, I found my family and friends staring at me with raised eyebrows in anticipation of hearing the doctor's news. My huge smile and relaxed body language must have given me away because their previously concerned faces now held smiles.

"He made it!" I yelled, throwing my fists into the air in victory.

They responded in claps, cheers, and "Thank you, Jesus!" We all hugged, and some of us shared of few tears of joy.

I said, "I'm fine now. You've been here long enough, so please go home. They'll be coming to get me soon."

They gathered their belongings, and each stopped in front of me to give me another hug or tell me they were glad Bob was okay. Seeing each of the faces and knowing the sacrifice they made with their time to support us demonstrated just how blessed we were.

I sat in the waiting room with my thoughts and prayers of thankfulness. Tick tock, tick tock, tick tock. I glanced at my watch—6:30 p.m. A whole hour had passed since Dr. Simpson came out to talk to me. Other families started leaving one by one, either to go home or be led back to recovery, until there was no one in the family waiting area but me.

The lady behind the desk said, "Mrs. Kormondy, I'm leaving now."

I scurried over to her and again asked (probably for the fifteenth time), "When can I go back to see Bob?"

She smiled and again responded (probably for the fifteenth time), "They still haven't called from recovery to let me know you can go back."

Disappointed, I returned to my seat. A few minutes later, the lights went off in the waiting area. Not only was I left all alone, but I was left alone in the dark. And I still hadn't been able to see my husband!

Everything felt all wrong. I rushed to the desk and picked up the phone to get some answers. I called and called for the next hour to no avail. When they turned off the lights, they must have turned off the heat as well. Anxious, cold, and afraid, I walked to the recovery room door, but it was locked.

It was like a ghost town, and I couldn't take it anymore. After pulling out my cell phone, I called the main operator for the hospital. "Can you please tell me what's going on? I'm up here in the family waiting area. The lights are out, and no one's answering the phone in recovery. My husband's been out of surgery for over two hours, but no one's come to get me. Was there an emergency with him? Did something go wrong? Is he all right? Please, I need a nurse to come out and tell me what's happening before I lose my mind."

In a professional monotone voice, the operator answered, "I'll send someone."

A few minutes later, her "someone" was a security guard. Although disappointed, I was thankful to speak to another human being.

"Ma'am, I checked to see what was happening. I was told that they were preparing to move him to the ICU and that you should go there."

Okay, something was happening. This was all very confusing, but I was getting closer to finding my husband.

I located the ICU and entered a huge area with rooms encircling the nurses' station. I must have looked as lost as I felt because a middle-aged nurse walked over to me. Her warm eyes and soft smile gave me some comfort.

"Can I help you?" she asked.

"Where's Bob Kormondy? I'm his wife Evelyn, and I was told that he was on the way up here from recovery."

"He's not up here yet, but I can take you to his room where you can wait for him," she offered.

I nodded and followed her to a clean room with all kinds of medical machines. "Thank you," I said and sat in the room's only chair.

After a few minutes, Bob had still not arrived. My heart began to pump quickly, and panic set in. *Where's Bob? I don't see him. He's supposed to be here.*

I rushed out of the room to find the nice nurse at the nurses' station and repeated my question to her. "Where's my husband? He's supposed to be here."

Her eyes softened in understanding. "It's okay, Mrs. Kormondy. Go back to his room and have a seat. I'll find out what's going on and then come and tell you."

After a few moments, she walked into the room. "I'm sorry, but we're showing your husband is still down in recovery, and they're not bringing him up yet." She pursed her lips and slightly shook her head. "They also said that he's been asking for his wife, but they told him she had gone home."

Devastated, I broke down in sobs. How could they tell him that? I had been in the waiting room the whole time, and no one called me to go back to him. Bob must have felt so alone thinking I had left him. How could they have been so heartless? How could they have cared so little that they didn't bother to check to see if I was there?

The whole time, I had tried to be calm and appreciative of what they were doing to help Bob; I didn't want to make any waves. Never again! Lesson learned! From here on, I would be Bob's advocate. I would be polite but not accepting of what was clearly a problem. This was a new environment, and *I* needed to change to adapt, and this adaptation started immediately!

−11−

Don't Leave

I ran out of the room and through the hospital until I came to an elevator and took it down to the recovery floor. My head was going to explode, but my hurt and anger propelled me until I got to my destination.

The door to the recovery room was locked. Mentally, I rolled my sleeves up and was ready to fight, which transferred to the physical—repeatedly banging on the recovery door with my fists and yelling, "Let me in! Let me in! Where's my husband? Let me in. I don't understand. I want to see my husband! What's happening? Somebody talk to me!"

Why hadn't I done this before? Why had I trusted them to look out for my husband's best interest? Look where that had gotten Bob . . . and me!

Finally, the door opened to a scowling nurse. "Stop banging on this door. What do you want?" he asked, his tone indignant.

"My husband's in there. His name's Bob Kormondy, and I want to see him *now*! I will *not* go away. Where is he?" I demanded in a tone that was just as indignant as his.

The nurse's eyebrows furrowed. "He's in here, but you have to calm down before you can come in."

I nodded and composed myself, wiping my face. He allowed me to enter. I was surprised at how dark the area was, but there was one source of light, and my eyes were instinctively drawn to it. In its midst was Bob looking so helpless lying in the only occupied bed. Tubes were coming out of his neck, or what was left of it.

I ran to his bed and gently bent over him. ""Honey, I'm here," I whispered.

A tear escaped from his eye and rolled down his cheek. He whispered back, "Where have you been?"

"I've been here the whole time trying to find you." Numerous tears fell from my eyes and unashamedly ran down my cheeks.

"Don't leave me," he pleaded.

My heart broke more. He seemed so helpless. "I'll be right here and hold you until we leave together," I assured him. "And then I'll remain by your side."

"Good. I need you. I didn't know it would hurt so much. Now the nurse is hurting me. He's been trying to force pills down my throat," he managed to say. "My throat hurts."

I couldn't believe it! He was in no condition to swallow anything after this invasive and radical neck and throat surgery, especially a hard pill. I couldn't help but wonder if this nurse was simply trying to complete his checklist so he could go home regardless of how it affected the patient. The new advocate in me reared up.

I walked over to the nurses' station and saw one man inputting something into a computer. "Are you Bob Kormondy's nurse?" I asked.

The man turned his head to contemplate me for a moment. "I am. Is there a problem?"

"Yes. Why are you trying to make him swallow pills?" I was now on the offensive. "Can't you see that he just had throat surgery? Why don't you give him a shot instead?"

The nurse shrugged. "He needs to just swallow his pills."

That was it! We were done with this narcistic nurse. "Take him to ICU! *Now!*" I demanded in a tone that told everyone in earshot that there was no negotiation.

We were moved and in the ICU within minutes.

Once there, the nurses set him up. They were so attentive and treated him with such kindness, a whole different world from what I had witnessed with the recovery room. They explained everything they did in detail. Thankfully, they gave him pain medication through an IV. Bob was more relaxed and started telling me what he remembered after the surgery.

He said, "My first recollection as soon as I woke up was *My goodness, does this hurt!* I knew they were going to do a lot to my throat, neck, and shoulder, but I really had no idea how painful it was going to be. I slept through most of my recovery. Then I woke up and looked for you, but no one was around my recovery bed. At that time, I didn't have a voice to call anyone. I could only make a tapping motion on the side of my gurney. It took a while for someone to show up. I could tell it was late, probably after normal hours because not a lot of staff were around. My throat hurt so bad, and I needed some kind of pain medication."

He paused for a moment. "The nurse came back with a pill for me to swallow. I told him I couldn't swallow a pill, to just give me a shot or some kind of liquid, but he insisted I swallow the pill. I also asked for you. He told me that no one was in the waiting room. I knew that couldn't be true. I asked him to please check again and bring you here."

"I must've fallen asleep because I woke up to the most wonderful voice saying, 'Honey, I'm here.' I'll never forget that sound, those words. I finally felt loved, safe, and secure. My love, my wonderful wife Evelyn, was here now. I knew everything was going to be okay."

My heart broke again. I held his hand and cried for what he went through, for what he would go through.

The next day, Dr. Simpson came to see Bob to remove the bandage. We became overwhelmed. We didn't realize just how brutal this surgery would be until the bandages were removed and we were able to see the staples down the side of Bob's neck and across his throat. We had never seen staples in a neck before, let alone so many.

Dr. Simpson noticed our surprise. "The cancer was very invasive. I was finding it in every direction I turned. It seemed like it just kept going, and I had to keep going too so I could make sure I got it all."

Not surprising, Dr. Simpson had done an excellent job. Thank God we were able to have a surgeon as talented and skilled as him.

I stayed with Bob the whole four days he was in ICU and slept in a recliner. The only time I left his side was to take a shower down the hall and to brush my teeth with the toothbrush and toothpaste the nurses had given me. Otherwise, no way was I going to leave him, leave that hospital, not until he came home and was safe in my arms.

It was challenging for Bob. He couldn't eat or drink, just slept. I kept the TV on low volume and watched the golf tournament he was supposed to be working in Naples, Florida at that time. When it aired, the announcer Dan Hicks did a shout out to Bob. Unfortunately, Bob was asleep and didn't see it live, but people from all over the country told him about it.

He also had numerous messages on his cell phone from colleagues and his network. It warmed his heart to know that he was missed and appreciated. They encouraged him, letting him know he would be welcomed back as soon as he recovered.

Those who sent these well wishes probably had no idea how wonderful their actions and words truly were. They bolstered Bob. In his eyes, I could see how they took him from his hospital bed in the ICU to the golf course where he could feel the breeze and hear the director's voice coming through his earpiece. And then with his camera on his shoulder, he would capture the great shot that had just been made.

These were invaluable gestures made that will never be forgotten by either of us!

After four days in the ICU, Bob got "promoted" (moved) to a regular room where he stayed for two days. I studied what the nurses did to take care of him, knowing that soon, that would be me.

The day he got discharged from the hospital, we were so happy! We couldn't wait to get home! It didn't matter what condition he was in; he was going home, and with the help of the Lord Jesus Christ, I could help him heal, do whatever was required.

I would now be Bob's nurse, and I embraced the challenge because no one on this planet had more passion, more motivation to ensure that he came through this ordeal successfully than me.

−12−

The Kormondy Medical Center

My world stopped, and nothing was as important as what was in front of me. It was all about Bob; he was all I cared about. I wanted to make sure he got the right medications at the right time, that he was comfortable, fed, and stayed encouraged. The doctors and nurses told me what to expect and what I would need to do to take care of him, and I intended to heed their advice to the letter.

So even before Bob's surgery, I made many adjustments in our house to accommodate his needs. Once we both came back home, I knew I would be running at full throttle.

My father had crafted for me a twelve-foot dining room table that sat sixteen. Perfect for a medical station. So I completely covered it with medical supplies and all of Bob's prescriptions.

Still, more room was needed, so I placed an additional table to the side to hold what the main table couldn't, like an appointment book and paperwork, including a typed chart for every medication, what it was for, possible side effects, the exact time to administer it, and the dosage amount. It also gave the time his bandages needed to be changed. Nothing could be forgotten in Bob's daily care, all critical for his recovery.

After reading and rereading the instructions, I still felt overwhelmed, but at least I knew everything Bob needed *before* he needed it. The tables were stacked high with no empty space, so I prayed for peace and calm in my head.

I clung to the thought that maybe when we're at the bottom of that stack and the table has less and less stuff on it, Bob would be getting better and better. Until then, my only job was to help save him, and along the way, I was to comfort him, love him, pray with him through this, and give him strength, even make him laugh.

Since his favorite place to sit in the family room was on the love seat, that would be perfect for his bed. So I brought out sheets and blankets and made it up. Then I put several different pillows around it.

The next challenge to address was Bob's eating and medication. The surgery had removed his salivary glands from the right side. Without saliva to lubricate his throat, it was difficult for him to swallow anything solid. Consequently, all of his food had to be pureed and his pills crushed to a powder and then mixed in with applesauce. Since I could no longer "cook" for him, I put that show of my love into the healthy concoctions I "created" for him from recipes that others had given us.

We both got a reprieve when we went to see Dr. Simpson two days after Bob's hospital discharge. He wanted to check on the staples. He also wanted to tell us what to expect in the near future.

"You'll need to call Dr. Martin's office," he stated. "If you recall, I had introduced him to you during our first exam. You'll be seeing him for radiation treatments. He's the best radiation oncologist, so make sure you do everything he tells you to do."

Bob sat silent, and I thought, *This man's been through so much already. Now he's gotta go through more? Can we just give him a break and some time to catch his breath?*

Then Dr. Simpson's words during his first visit flooded through my brain—four months to live.

"When does he need to start radiation?" I asked.

Dr. Simpson's eyes darted back and forth between Bob and me. "As soon as possible. I know we're upon the holidays, but I suggest you go ahead and call and make an appointment now."

I nodded as I watched Bob, hoping for some reaction. I didn't get any.

We drove home, or back to our new "medical center." Apparently, there was still a lot ahead of us, and we had only begun this journey. Bob's vocal cord cancer was not as serious as his neck and throat cancer, so no chemotherapy or radiation was needed. Same with my previous cancer, and they were all I had to compare his journey to. Despite all my preplanning and organization, I had been thrown into an area I really knew nothing about and was flying by the seat of my pants.

By the time we got home from our appointment with Dr. Simpson, we were both down and lost in our own thoughts. Then we heard our doorbell ringing.

I looked out the peephole and saw a delivery man

holding a large and oddly shaped package. I opened the door.

"May I help you?" I asked.

"Yeah. Got a package for Robert Kormondy from a Francisco Goya," he read in a happy-go-lucky tone from the shipping label.

"Bob!" I yelled over my shoulder. "Francisco Goya sent you a package."

Francisco Goya was Bob's friend and world-class windsurfing champion from Maui.

Then I turned back to the delivery man. "Can you bring it in for us and put it over there on our living room floor?"

"Sure," he answered.

I stepped aside as the delivery man walked in with the box. About that same time, Bob hobbled into the room, his eyes glued on the box.

"Wow!" he exclaimed.

We thanked the delivery man, and he left. Bob and I were excited and curious, although I was not as excited as him but probably just as intrigued.

I got a box cutter to slice through the tape and peel back the cardboard flaps. Inside revealed a gorgeous windsurfing board. On top was a handwritten note from Francisco telling Bob to recover soon and get back into the sport of windsurfing.

Bob's grin covered his face as he ran his hand over the smooth texture of the board. "I can't wait to get out there with this," he commented in a dreamy voice.

Francisco's timing was perfect. This was just what Bob needed to put some positive back into his life and to let him see the future and motivate him. Mostly, it was what he needed at that time to realize that other people were in this fight with him, even if they were on the other side of the world.

Soon after receiving Francisco's gift, things began to turn around. Our efforts seemed to be working. After a week, Bob told me he felt rather normal. He said that his mouth felt better, and he didn't feel any pain. Even better, the remaining salivary glands were producing saliva now.

We both chuckled over this phenomenon because saliva wasn't something we had ever really thought about. Now we recognized it to be a really wonderful thing, and I celebrated this reclaimed gift with him.

However, another unfortunate side effect of throat

surgery that Bob and I hadn't considered to this point was the beard growing around certain areas on his neck. It caused him discomfort and got rather itchy. If nothing was done and done soon, I could see it getting out of control. However, I was afraid if I tried to shave him. I might mess up his staples . . . or worse.

I called my mom to tell her about our dilemma. She then called Eula, her hairdresser for thirty years. Of course, Eula came right over along with my mom and my sister Patty. My mom sat on the couch and encouraged Bob as the rest of us surrounded him to start the task that would make him more comfortable.

He took in a deep breath and let us work. I held his face, and my friend held his head while Eula used a straight razor on all his stubble, even on his neck.

My mother's reward for having such a wonderful idea was her enjoyment in watching us try to handle such a task. She would add a little fun to our new venture, chuckling now and then as we fumbled through it. Looking back, I guess we must have been a funny sight.

And then, it was over! Thank God for Eula! She made what seemed to be an unsurmountable task successful.

Afterwards, Bob looked around at all of us with a contented smile. "Thank you," he said. "I feel so much better. Plus, it's nice to be surrounded by all these women."

This venture was such a success that we decided we would do it again. I didn't know if I could ever be comfortable shaving his face with staples. So as long as Eula was willing, we would wait until he really needed another shave to contact her for another round. She assured me she would return.

Bob's freshly shaven face helped bring a little normalcy to an abnormal situation. He was improving but under the watchful eye and scrutiny of Dr. Simpson. We became "frequent flyers" to his office because he needed to check on the progress of Bob's staples often so that at some point, he could take them out.

Finally, about two to three weeks postoperatively, Dr. Simpson felt confident that enough healing had taken place to remove them. Bob was so ready; he really wanted them out. Despite Eula's shaves, the itching was increasing as the healing increased. But the process actually turned out to be a very painful experience with the pull of each staple. Once out, though, he had even more relief.

In addition to the visual check-ins, he also underwent a lot of bloodwork to monitor the results, including his white and red blood cell counts.

Soon afterward, Bob signed up for a scientific study that required him to do additional bloodwork so that others like him would hopefully be helped in the future. He wanted to prevent them from going through what he did. But that was who Bob was—always thinking of others.

What an amazing Christian man I married!

– 13 –

Who Knew About the Teeth

Three days before Christmas 2011, we had an appointment with Dr. Matt Lewis, a specialty dentist. Both Bob's and my dentists had referred us to him. They knew Bob was going through radiation for throat cancer, and he had a few teeth with some decay. Infection was a concern, but they wouldn't have time to fix them before radiation started. As a result, they needed to be pulled.

Evidently, radiation is exceptionally hard on the mouth and can cause teeth to fall out anyway. Dr. Lewis had us make this appointment so that before he extracted those few teeth, he could make impressions of them to replace them at a later date.

We ended up staying so busy with medical appointments that if not for all the festive decorations and colorful lights, I would have forgotten it was the Christmas season, my favorite time of year. I'm like a little girl during this particular holiday, and Bob and I always decorated quite a bit together.

Since that wasn't possible this year, my dad came over to help. We decorated the family room where Bob stayed, including putting the Christmas tree in there and decorating it as well so that Bob could enjoy it.

The rest of the house didn't have any decorations; it continued to look like a hospital, but at least it looked like a warm and welcoming hospital. It had no institutional colors. Instead, my home decorating touches and the pictures I had shot were framed and strategically placed everywhere to give it that friendly and comfortable ambiance.

The girls came to visit, and we all spent a quiet Christmas Eve together watching Christmas movies, such as *It's a Wonderful Life*. The girls took turns snuggling with their dad and loving on him, and I enjoyed sitting on the couch with the other two.

My mom and dad showed up the next morning, as always. The family was now all here, and Christmas turned out to be absolutely wonderful. I cooked breakfast while the three girls talked to their dad, with the youngest, Charlene, snuggled up on the couch beside him. The togetherness during this trying time made me love my family even more. We laughed and bonded, and I felt truly blessed.

And then Christmas was over. Everyone left to go back to their own homes and lives, back to reality, and the fairytale ended.

Two days later on December 27, we returned to Dr. Lewis. We were up against a tight deadline, knowing that soon, radiation would begin. Now that he had made molds for the unfortunate teeth, time to extract them. It all had to be done prior to Bob undergoing radiation.

All of this was just in time to welcome in 2012. We were heading into a new year. When we were younger, Bob and I went out to a lot of New Year's Eve events and celebrated. But this year, we stayed home. Frankly, we were flat-out tired! We had more activity in the past six weeks than we had for the whole year.

So 2011 ended without further ado. We cuddled together on the love seat to watch the countdown, but we both fell asleep before it began.

In the wee hours that morning, we woke up and realized we had missed the whole countdown. We laughed.

Bob said, "Oh, it's 2012."

I nodded in agreement. "It's going to be an amazing year, Bob, blessed by our Lord and Savior!"

– 14 –

The Plan to Survive

It was still dark outside as we drove west to the hospital for Bob's first appointment with his radiation oncologist, Dr. Martin. We were only two days into the week and three days into 2012, and my head was spinning with everything that had to be done.

The early morning appointment reminded me of driving to Bob's surgery just a few weeks ago. Our hopes were high that maybe this wouldn't be as brutal.

Bob was strong and approached everything that came his way with the attitude of "We'll take it as it comes, Evie; it's the way we are. Just get through what we need to do for today and not worry about tomorrow; that's on the calendar where it belongs. It's not as if we can do any more than we're already doing to take care of today."

Neither one of us knew what to expect. Although we both had gone through and survived cancer, we had never known anyone to go through this type of throat cancer radiation.

The visit started out on a good foot with Dr. Martin's nurse. Her bright and cheery voice reverberated in the waiting room as she called Bob back to the exam rooms.

As we approached her, the smile on her face didn't disappoint. She turned out to be a genuinely nice person. Granted, we were a little nervous as she led us to the small exam room. She asked a few questions and then announced, "Dr. Martin will be with you momentarily."

We waited for the doctor for what seemed like a long time. Left alone, we talked about what we thought would happen next, but it was all speculation. And we prayed.

Finally, Dr. Martin walked in. He had fair skin and strawberry-blond hair. His smile was warm as he held his hand out for Bob to shake.

"Hi Bob," he said in a strong voice. "I'm Dr. Martin."

After some small talk, Dr. Martin got down to business. I appreciated his mannerism—extremely nice and confident—as he explained to us what was ahead for

Bob, the radiation plan and treatments, what to expect, and what we needed to do.

"We've got your first radiation treatment scheduled for January 17 at 8 a.m." He flipped through the notes on a clipboard.

"That's in less than two weeks," I blurted out.

Dr. Martin glanced from his clipboard to my surprised face and waited for me to continue. When I didn't, he said, "It looks like you'll have a second treatment that same day at 2:00. Your treatments will take place every weekday, Monday through Friday, at 8 a.m. and 2 p.m. for a total of thirty-two days, five and a half weeks. Your last one will be on Tuesday, March 1. And . . . you cannot miss one treatment. We'll do periodic CT scans to check the progress of both the radiation and the surgery and their success in shrinking any cancer and tumors that weren't found in the surgery."

I spoke again, this time sharing the fast math I was doing in my head. "Twice a day for thirty-two days? So that's sixty-four treatments in all? Isn't that a lot?"

Dr. Martin nodded his head. "Yes, it is. It's actually a near-unheard of amount of radiation, but we have to be more aggressive than the cancer."

Taking in a deep breath, I raised my eyebrows. Our hopes that the surgery was the biggest part of his treatment and that this was backup had just been dashed. The opponent was much stronger than we thought, so the fight was still on.

Thinking about Bob's lifestyle, I said, "Bob is very active. He surfs and is always participating in some type of sports. How will this affect him?"

Dr. Martin pursed his lips. "Yes, I've seen that in Bob's records, that he was very active in sports. I'm sorry, but Bob does need to prepare himself because he won't be able to surf or engage in sports again."

Watching Bob's reaction, the pain in his eyes, this ominous prognosis had cut him to the core. I was very angry with the doctor for making such a negative declaration. He didn't know anything with certainty, only God did, and God knew Bob and his strength and how hard he would work to get his life back. Why take everything away that gives him strength and hope as he entered what apparently was going to be a very dark place?

Then my anger calmed as I realized the doctor had just seen too much darkness and was probably laying out the worst possible outcome. After all, we did need to know what Bob was facing. The doctor had no idea we had a vast support team in place—God, Bob, our family, our friends, our church, prayer circles, and me all pulling together for Bob's full recovery.

I envisioned Bob driving east and finding a way to surf. His recovery didn't need to be textbook perfect; it would be perfect enough for him to hit the water and get out past the breakers.

I could see it so clearly in my mind's eye. For sure, it would happen!

Bob finally spoke up. "I have a question. Do I really need radiation? Can we just wait to see if it's necessary?"

The doctor paused and stared directly into his eyes. "Well," he started, his voice firm, "It was nice knowing you, son."

What was that supposed to mean? Was he so offended by Bob's question that he didn't want to treat him? Was this his way of saying, "Bye-bye; have a good life"? Or did it mean that if Bob didn't have the radiation treatments, then he wouldn't need Dr. Martin's services since radiation treatments were what he did?

That was a confusing statement, and I needed clarity. So I asked, "What does that mean?"

He now directed his gaze onto me. "Bob won't survive if we don't do everything possible now, everything that we can do to eradicate this cancer . . . now. He won't have the opportunity to see if it's necessary. It's necessary now, and if he thinks he can wait, plain and simple, he'll die in less than four months."

There was that "four months expiration date" again. Our minds were blown. We again looked at each other, neither knowing how to respond.

"Can we have a moment please?" I requested.

"Sure," the doctor answered.

After he and his assistant left the room, Bob and I prayed. We talked to the Lord and asked Him for direction and guidance. We then talked to each other and decided that together, we could go through the radiation. Really, Bob had to go through it all. I was there just to hold his hand. Thank God, he was so strong.

By the time Dr. Martin returned, we felt confident with our decision.

"Dr. Martin," Bob started, glancing over to me

momentarily, "I'll do the radiation."

The doctor gave a nod in agreement. "Great! We need to get started right away then. Here's the schedule we've put together for your treatments."

The nurse handed us a sheet of paper that was full of dates, sixty-four in all. The busy life we lived before seemed like one of idleness compared to what we had in front of us.

Dr. Martin added, "While you are here, we need to fit you with the mask."

Bob's eyes danced in mischievousness as he looked as me. "Oh yeah? What's that about? Sounds like it could add some fun."

His comment took me by surprise, but it was a good surprise. Bob must have resigned himself to going through the radiation and was trying to find the positive in what laid ahead. Consequently, the atmosphere immediately switched from heavy to light.

The doctor explained, "The mask is for you to wear during radiation. It'll have holes so that we can track exactly where the radiation goes each time. The mask will go over your face and neck and be attached to the table to keep your head from moving and twitching during the treatment. It's crucial that the radiation is applied to the exact location needed."

The whole mask thing actually scared me. It sounded restraining and smothering. I didn't want to dash Bob's attempts at positivity, so I just smiled in an effort to encourage him.

Bob followed the doctor down the hallway to get fitted for the mask, and I headed back to the waiting room as instructed. Thinking about that mask and how Bob's head would be strapped to a table put me into a bit of a panic attack. I prayed that God would give me peace and calm so that I would be there for my husband. I loved him so much, and I wanted to add to his strength and be optimistic every step of the way.

Heading east to go home was always uplifting to us, but that day, Bob was fairly quiet. The long appointment gave us more information than we really wanted, even though we knew we needed the facts. Sometimes the facts are harder to take than you anticipated, or they're simply not the facts you had hoped to hear.

That night, Bob finally talked about the mask. "Actually, I found getting fitted for it somewhat fascinating. I've played hockey, so I can relate to having to wear a mask even though I never played goalie. It's going to be a new experience, Evie, but mostly, like a goalie's mask, this mask will protect me. It's gonna make sure that the radiation hits the exact spot, and hopefully, the radiation will do exactly what is needed with as little damage as possible."

I smiled but didn't respond, afraid that I would reveal my fear. I was not going to do anything except reinforce his positive attitude.

Bob studied my face. He must not have bought into my attempts at reinforcement because he tried to reassure me it would be fine. "Evie, don't worry. I'll be able to breathe easily through the mask. It'll be fun putting it on and seeing how it works."

He was more courageous than me. From the time we were first together, one of the traits I had so admired about him was his calmness and quiet strength throughout whatever was going on at the time in our lives. To me, this cancer was so much bigger than anything we had ever faced, and his attitude and strength awed me.

I prayed for God to stay beside him every step of the way, to help him endure what might be more difficult than he thought, and to help me say and do just what was needed to support him through the coming weeks.

But before we had a chance to process the impending radiation schedule, Bob had to undergo more bloodwork, and we had an appointment two days later with Dr. Brock, Bob's chemotherapy doctor. Like Dr. Martin did with Bob's radiation, Dr. Brock had gone ahead and set up Bob's chemotherapy schedule.

"You'll have a total of seven treatments with your first on January 18 and then again on January 25, 27, and February 3, 8, 15, and the last on February 22," he explained.

Seven treatments sounded a whole lot better than the sixty-four scheduled for radiation. Still . . .

"But he'll also be undergoing radiation two times a day starting on January 17," I notified him.

He nodded. "Yes, I'm aware of his radiation schedule. However, we also need to start chemo as soon as possible, and we can't wait until he completes his radiation treatments. So on the days he is scheduled for both, the chemotherapy will need to take place after the morning radiation treatment."

I nodded in understanding, although I wasn't sure I understood any of it.

Dear God, I silently prayed, *how much more can one man take? Please help Bob."*

– 15 –

Financial Hardship

Five days before Bob's treatments were to begin, we celebrated our tenth anniversary on January 12. Again, just like New Year's Eve, we made the evening low-key, choosing to simply be together.

We talked about how blessed we were to have found each other and how much we loved each other, and no matter what, we would always be with each other forever. Then we popped in a good movie and fell asleep on the couch holding hands.

The next day was back to reality. Seeing some of what laid ahead, I realized that neither Bob nor I would be bringing in much income, yet we still had bills. We were both independent contractors, so if we didn't work, we didn't get paid. In fact, we hadn't worked for the last month, and we would definitely not be able to work for the next two months while Bob underwent these treatments. They would not only keep us busy—a full-time job for both of us—but I anticipated that Bob would experience some negative side effects that would render him almost incapacitated.

Furthermore, we didn't have any vacation time or sick leave, nor did we have any supplemental insurance policies. We only had our savings to fall back on, and that was not unlimited.

I vacillated as to if I should discuss these financial woes with Bob at the time. The last thing I needed to do was dump more stress on him. Therefore, I decided I would handle it by myself. I was a big girl, and I knew Bob trusted my judgement.

The biggest bill we had was our mortgage, so I called our mortgage lender. We had been long-time customers and had always paid our mortgage early and paid more than the payment due amount.

I spoke to the representative and told her about Bob, what occurred with him last month, and what was scheduled for him over the next couple of months. "We've been with this mortgage company for a really long time," I reminded her. "Can you work with us during this period when we simply can't pay our mortgage?"

The representative responded in an understanding and empathetic tone. "I am so sorry to hear all that's happening to you and your husband, Mrs. Kormondy. I can see that you've been a valuable customer, so sure, we can help. We can offer you a hardship refinance where we defer your mortgage for a year with no fees. Until you get approved for this hardship refinance, I can set you up so that you won't have a mortgage payment until May 1."

"Thank you! That will surely help. Is there anything I need to do in the meantime?" I asked, wanting as much clarity as possible. This was our home we were talking about, so I wanted to make sure I didn't miss a thing.

"Yes. Just don't make any payments during this month. It'll confuse the refinance process," she stated with confidence and conviction.

Paying nothing was hard for me to wrap my head around. "So you're saying that even if I can pay something toward my mortgage, I shouldn't?"

"That's right. Do not send us any money. You'll be just fine. I'll let you know when we've finished the refinance paperwork. In the meantime, we'll be mailing you a package with all the information. Make sure you read through it and understand it," she instructed.

A few days later, I received the package from our mortgage lender. It explained they were working on a hardship refinance for us, and it gave the terms.

Still, I put it on my calendar to call every week to follow up with the representative and the status of the refinance. Each time, I would check to see if I needed to do anything. I would even ask, "Do I need to try to raise the money for our monthly mortgage until all of this is settled?"

Losing our house for lack of payment was not what we needed at this time . . . really, not at any time.

The representative would say, "No. You and your husband have a wonderful standing with us. If you make a payment, it'll mess up the process and progress of the refinance."

I trusted her and that she knew what she was doing and was looking out for us. Honestly, I was so busy taking care of Bob that it was a relief to have someone else taking this burden off my plate. It allowed me to put my focus where it was needed.

One challenge down, but we had many more to go.

– 16 –

The Mask of Precision

The night before Bob's first radiation treatment, I hardly slept because I felt like I couldn't breathe. Glancing over at the alarm clock, it was only a few minutes until the alarm clock went off anyway, so I quietly got up and onto my knees. I needed to be light, positive, and courageous, all of which seemed beyond my reach at that moment.

I prayed, "God, help Bob through this most difficult time, and give me strength to match his. Please, please calm my fears."

Bob woke up in an optimistic mood. It was hard keeping up with his cheery demeanor, but I tried to match his same tone nevertheless. We agreed that by going ahead and getting started on these treatments, he would get them done and over with that much sooner.

The night before, he had told me, "Evie, I feel strong and that I can take just about anything."

Yet neither of us knew what that "anything" looked like during these radiation treatments. Undoubtedly, Bob was mentally strong and physically stronger than he had been just a few weeks ago when he was recovering from major surgery. He now seemed to be as ready as he would ever be.

One step at a time. Just handle today. Tomorrow will take care of itself. Clichés and our motto kept inundating my mind, but to us, they never lost meaning; they were very much front and center.

Despite Jacksonville's horrid rush-hour traffic that morning, we showed up at Mercy Hospital early, ready to fight this cancer. Within minutes of arriving, they called Bob back to change into a hospital gown before directing him to a sterile and cold treatment room that contained a sterile and cold table. At least the staff was warm as they greeted us.

A young man in his early thirties instructed Bob to climb up on that sterile and cold table and lie back. He complied, and the man draped the mask over and around Bob's face and entire neck. Then he proceeded to screw the edges of the mask into the table.

I stood over to the side against the wall, far enough

away to give them the space to work on Bob but close enough to see the tear coming out of his eye during the drilling process.

A knife cut through my heart as I saw my husband strapped down to that table and constrained from the neck up. Inside my head, I screamed, *What are you doing? Stop it! Set my husband free!*

I was so glad that Bob couldn't see my tears as I wept in the shadows of the room. I understood the purpose, but it didn't lessen the emotional pain.

Bob kept saying, "I'm okay, Evie."

There he was with his head screwed to a table, yet he was encouraging me. No matter how many times he tried, it didn't take away the horrible sight of what they were doing to him. It was like watching something out of a scary movie.

The staff told us that everyone had to leave the room during the treatment. I hated to go, feeling so helpless and like I was abandoning my husband in this condition.

"Sweetheart," I said, trying to keep my voice from cracking, "this will be over in a few minutes. I'm just gonna step out of the room, and the Lord Jesus is going to be in here with you, holding you as you go through this. You are not alone."

"I'm okay, Evie," he repeated through the mask.

I glanced over my shoulder and saw another tear rolling out of the corner of Bob's eye and down his face. The sweet nurse wiped it away, but it still choked me up again.

We all walked out of the room. A middle-aged man with glasses talked to him over the speaker. "Mr. Kormondy, what kind of music do you like?"

"Alan Jackson or Jimmy Buffet would be great," Bob answered.

Within moments, Jimmy Buffet resounded throughout the treatment room. "Can you hear the music okay?" the middle-aged man asked.

"Yes," Bob answered, sounding less stressed.

The middle-aged man said, "We'll let you know when we'll be starting and stopping."

The nurse turned to me and said, "You can go back to the waiting room."

I hesitated as I tried to process her words. It was hard enough to leave him in that room by himself, and now I had to be farther away in the waiting room?

I didn't argue, but I did ask, "Can you come and get me when he gets dressed?"

She smiled. "I can do that."

Sitting in that waiting room was very stressful as I thought about the machine in another room sending radiation through Bob's neck. Even though the actual radiation time was about forty minutes, I had no idea how long he would be back there.

After what seemed like forever, a nurse called me to go back with her. "He's all done. Follow me."

By the time I got to the dressing room, he was almost dressed, just buttoning his shirt. He looked just like he did before the treatment. I didn't know what I was expecting, maybe that he would be drained and look weak, but this was good; no, this was great!

We left to go home and headed east, but we only had a few hours before we had to return, just enough time for Bob to rest in the La-Z-Boy recliner and have a little to eat. Time sped by, and then we were in the car and driving back to the treatment center for another round. By 3:30 p.m., we were back home again for the rest of the day.

As I got Bob situated on the loveseat, I asked, "Are you feeling okay?"

He nodded. "Yes, I feel fine. It was interesting, though. As I lay on the radiation table with the mask over my face, I thought, *Wow, this is kind of a neat experience.* I was trying to be positive. I like the medical team working in that radiation room; they're friendly even though they knew my throat was about to be brutalized. The music I chose helped; it soothed me. Right now, I'm not noticing a difference, but from what I understand, radiation's cumulative. I'm told that for the first few weeks, I should be feeling okay."

So far, so good. I walked over to my calendar and marked the date off. One day of radiation down, thirty-one to go.

But then day two was more time-consuming as the chemotherapy was added to an already-crazy day consisting of two radiation treatments. The nurse had Bob sit in a recliner-like chair next to an IV pole with bags of chemotherapy fluids hanging from it. Tubes ran from the bags to Bob so the chemo could be infused into his body.

By the end of the day, not only was Bob understandably exhausted, but he got sick from the chemotherapy, something we anticipated because of the stories we had heard from others who had taken it. Bob didn't complain, though. However, I could hear him getting sick in the bathroom, and he wanted to be left alone.

He was also bored. Although he remained positive, he couldn't partake in the active lifestyle he had become accustomed to. Instead, he sat in a car going back and forth to the hospital twice a day for radiation, and then every few days, chemo treatment would be added.

I guess we could have stayed on that side of town on those three-treatment days, but home was our sanctuary. If Bob only had ten minutes to get away from it all, then we would have.

We took every day as it came. When each one ended, I received the satisfaction of marking it off the calendar. Weekends consisted of Bob resting, but they sped by. On Sunday nights, apprehension hovered over us as we recognized we were heading into another week of chemicals and burns.

For the first eight days of treatments, Bob started wondering if the radiation was doing any good. "I don't feel anything happening," he stated. "These treatments are a waste."

We were hoping that the inevitable wouldn't affect

Bob like those who had gone before him. We could hope, but deep inside, we knew it was a just matter of time.

–17–

God's Gift of a Second Chance

Bob's oncologist, Dr. Brock, moved on at the end of January, and a new doctor took his place. It turned out that this new chemo doctor, Dr. Jim Davis, was not a stranger to us. He was our neighbor, our friend, and Bob's archery partner. Small world. One could say it was quite the coincidence, but I trust the God of "coincidences," a God who had laid out Bob's journey before He formed him in his mother's womb (Jeremiah 1:5).

In fact, nothing we went through was by circumstance but divinely orchestrated by the Almighty. Dr. Davis was a prime example.

So let me give the back story to our relationship with Dr. Davis. A few months before Bob's diagnosis, I learned that a new family—a nice couple with two children—had moved into our neighborhood. The Friday after Bob's initial appointment with Dr. Tucker, I baked a lemon cake and took it to them to introduce myself and welcome them to the neighborhood.

I really liked the wife and decided I would like to get to know her better. So, I asked her if she and her family could come to our house for dinner that Saturday night.

She accepted, and we met her husband Jim and their two daughters and got to know them better. They got to know us better too.

We learned that Jim was a medical doctor. At that time, we had no idea that Bob had cancer, so we didn't ask what kind of doctor he was, nor did he specify.

During dinner, Jim seemed to frequently glance at Bob's neck. Afterwards when his daughters left the room, he shared his concerns about the swelling that he had observed.

Bob shrugged it off as no big deal. "I went to an ear, nose, and throat doctor yesterday. He ran a few tests and said he'd have the results when we get back from Australia."

We told the Davises about our Australia plans, but Jim continued to have a look of concern throughout that conversation. Then they moved on to talk about sports and found out that they shared a lot of interests. That night, Bob and I gained new friends, but the friendship grew stronger between the two men as time went on.

Knowing Dr. Jim Davis on a personal level was one thing, but now we got to see him on a professional level. As Bob's new oncologist, he had been assigned to help save my husband.

While in his office, our relationship was different. He was no longer "Jim," but we respected his role and referred to him as "Dr. Davis."

We were just as impressed with his competence as a doctor as we were with his loyalty as a friend. He had a wonderful bedside manner, demonstrating kindness and intelligence as he shared his treatment plan for Bob. We left there that day feeling confident in his hands.

And then one night, our confidence in his ability was tested . . .

Bob had not been feeling well and didn't want dinner. Then as it got later, he decided to have a little something. As he was finishing his small meal, he couldn't swallow; his throat was closing. I gave him Swish (a medication used to treat mouth and throat discomfort), but it didn't help. I was scared he wasn't going to be able to breathe. Because it was so late at night, I considered calling 911.

Then an idea popped into my mind. As calmly as possible, I said, "Bob, I'll be right back."

Without taking the time to put on my shoes, I ran out the front door in my bare feet and didn't stop until I reached the Davises' house. Because I was in such a panic, I didn't even think about calling first.

I banged on their door as hard as I could. The ruckus may have woken up some close-by neighbors, but that was the least of my problems, so I kept pounding.

Finally, the porch light came on, and the door opened. Jim stood looking tired. I hoped I hadn't woken him up, but he would forgive me once he found out why I did.

I blurted out, "Bob's in trouble. He can't swallow, and his throat's closing. I'm scared he's not able to breathe!"

"Wait here," he instructed. Within seconds, he was back with a small bottle of something in his hand, and we both ran as fast as we could to my house.

When we arrived, Bob was still struggling to breathe. Jim quickly assessed the situation and sprayed whatever was in that bottle onto Bob's throat. Immediately, Bob drew in a gulp of air and was able to breathe again.

And so did I after seeing he was going to be okay.

Jim said, "Evelyn, I'm glad you came to get me. Bob wouldn't have made it if you had called 911. By the time they got here, it would've been too late."

Without a doubt, Dr. Jim Davis was an answer to our prayers, a gift from God, and a powerful testament that in the midst of our trials, He had our back and was with us.

– 18 –

Feeding the Feeding Tube

By January 30, Bob had undergone twenty radiation treatments and three chemotherapy treatments. Throughout this period, he could only eat small amounts of food at a time, and this was not doing the job of nourishing him. His weight was dropping rapidly. He had been in really good shape, doing whatever physical activity he wanted to do, but now, he was thin and weak.

The chemo and radiation treatments were taking a toll on him. In particular, we started witnessing the cumulative effects of radiation rearing its ugly head. Those last two treatments on Friday, January 28 were likened to a cup that had filled up and now overflowed as his body seemed to buckle under the radiation's overbearing vengeance. It became too painful for him to eat at all, and he could barely get down any water.

Bob told me that it hurt worse on the inside of his throat than on the outside. The outside was like a bad sunburn and destroyed the skin, but on the inside, the radiation damaged the esophagus and destroyed the only salivary glands he had left after his surgery.

Dr. Martin had given him a prescription for a swish and swallow solution, which was a concoction to numb his throat between treatments and help him eat and drink as well as prevent his throat from getting an infection. For a while, that was the only way he could tolerate the pain, but it wasn't working anymore.

Bob was five foot eleven inches tall. Before the surgery, he weighed 195 pounds. In the seven weeks since then, he had lost forty-seven pounds and was now down to weighing 148. We were all scared. He wasn't even halfway through the radiation treatments, and none of us forgot that the effects were cumulative. We couldn't even imagine what the coming days would bring.

He couldn't keep going and sustain life without intervention. As a result, Dr. Martin announced that on Monday, February 6, Bob would be getting a feeding tube inserted. But the radiation would need to continue;

they could not stop. Nothing deterred the treatments. It seemed that they would never stop . . . never!

We were glad when that Monday came, even though we knew it was going to be a tough day—one surgery and two rounds of radiation. We were both eager to get his morning and afternoon treatments over with because Bob was actually looking forward to having the feeding tube.

But it required surgery to implant it. At this point, though, Bob didn't care. We had been able to talk with others beforehand who had gone through this procedure, and they eased our minds as to what to expect with the surgery.

Some people may think that having a feeding tube inserted was a bad thing, but we looked at it as a blessing. The bad thing was trying to eat when you couldn't but knowing you needed food. The good thing was having a device that would get the nutrients down so you didn't starve to death. We prayed together that all would go well.

So around 3:00 p.m. that day, right after his last treatment, we left that building and walked to the outpatient surgery center.

God again answered our prayers. Bob came out of the surgery fine, no surprises; everything happened as we had been told.

Like everything else thus far, we didn't think a feeding tube would be a big deal, and like most everything else thus far, it turned out to be huge. The surgery was the easy part, but we were learning that living with a feeding tube day-in and day-out was anything but.

First of all, Bob needed nutrition, and Ensure was the best choice. His social worker gave us a few cases. At first, Bob thought it was fun, pouring fluids into a funnel and hearing a gurgle in his belly. But then it became overwhelming. Pouring in a can of Ensure every two hours and then water every other hour in between—well, his stomach could only hold so much because it was shrinking.

The next challenge was the short length of time it took before we ran out of Ensure, and it was expensive. I was forced to become resourceful and called Abbott Nutrition, the company that owns Ensure. After all, I had nothing to lose and everything to gain.

I told them about Bob's situation. Five days later, seven cases with twelve cans each arrived, and we didn't have to pay a dime! What a blessing! There would be enough Ensure to last about twenty-one days!

Thank You, God, that You love us so much to make sure our needs are met!

In addition to Bob's nutrition, his lack of salivary glands caused him to need other products. His inability to produce any moisture in his mouth was painful, and he couldn't swallow. We were told how the product Biotene was fantastic in that it helped a lot with dry mouth. It was super expensive in the stores, and we simply didn't have the money to purchase it, even though it would have been worth every penny.

So I contacted the Biotene company as well. I spoke to a very nice woman and described Bob's situation.

She said, "I'm sorry to hear this. Tell you what. I'll send you a care kit that will include all of Biotene's products that help with dry mouth."

Sure enough, within a few days, Bob's care kit arrived. It contained a swish and swallow product and a special gum and toothpaste, the latter of which Bob uses to this day.

I also reached out via an email to a company that sold coconut water. Coconut water has a lot of health benefits, including being a great source of hydration. The company responded about a week later and sent a couple of free cases of it.

I learned that a lot of companies out there will help, but I had to ask. I was so glad we had a case manager who assisted us in navigating the process and performed wonders. For a cancer victim, case managers are a must and a crucial part of the process.

Bob no longer knew what taste was or even what hunger was. Desperate to get nutrition into Bob, I would make up a lot of different healthy drinks to pour into his feeding tube. We tried different things and discovered what worked and what upset his stomach somewhat or wouldn't go down the tube.

We learned that if Bob didn't have something in his stomach at all times, even if it was only water or an energy drink, it would try to ingest the feeding tube's ball that kept it in place. It was weird to think that a person's stomach actively searches for food when it's hungry.

At first, Bob thought feeling your stomach pull at the little ball was a neat sensation, but after a while, it started to hurt. Several times, he had to go back to the hospital and have his feeding tube adjusted.

It was worth it, though. He would no longer have to try to force a miniscule amount of food down his throat that now had an opening one tenth the size of a marble. He was able to finally feed his body and get more nutrition into his stomach.

Then one day, my sister Maria and her husband Ed came to visit. She had cancer when she was in her twenties, but thankfully, she had survived it. As a result of her experience, she became incredibly healthy and watched everything she ate. Maria would constantly teach us about healthy eating as she wanted to share her newfound wealth of nutritional knowledge.

We were all in the family room when Maria stood up and walked into the kitchen. She stepped into the pantry and surveyed its contents. After a few moments of silence, she came back out.

"Okay, I'm going to make you two healthy," she announced in the cutest Southern accent and with the biggest smile on her face. "And there isn't anything you can do about it."

Bob and I glanced at each other in confusion.

After her speech, she walked back into the pantry.

"Hey, Ed," she yelled in her accent, "bring the garbage can over here."

"Why do you need the garbage can, Maria?" I asked.

"Because your pantry is full of death. We have to throw out all this bad food."

Bob piped in, defending our pantry contents. "Maria, don't throw out my potato chips. I love my potato chips."

"Bob, you have a feeding tube. You can't even eat potato chips. All these things in here are unhealthy. They are so bad for you, so we have to get rid of all of them," Maria spouted matter-of-factly.

So she went to work getting rid of all the bad food by tossing them in the trash. She made us laugh because she was determined that we were going to learn to eat healthy. And we did! Thank you, Maria.

– 19 –

A Shot in the Arm

Bob had become severely dehydrated, but the feeding tube couldn't accept enough liquids to keep him hydrated enough. So IV fluids were ordered.

Thank God Dr. Martin ordered home healthcare to go with the IVs! When their nurse arrived at our house, I was so glad to see her. She was Irish, probably in her fifties, and introduced herself as "Mary."

Mary was one of those people who was easy to love. She would become a welcome sight every time she came to our house. Her assistance, insight, and intelligence helped tremendously with overwhelming tasks during an overwhelming time.

During that first visit, Mary explained everything in detail regarding what she was there to do and how she was going to do it. We found her to be warm, gentle, and experienced . . . just overall amazing!

I had so many questions, and she gave me even

more answers to questions I didn't yet know I had. With an endless supply of patience, she taught me and guided me in figuring out a lot of things in caring for Bob. But before that visit was over, I found out she still had a whole lot more to teach me—well, what felt like a whole lot more to me.

"Ms. Evelyn, now that your husband is on a feeding tube, I need to teach you how to give him his daily IVs."

My eyes popped wide open while my jaw dropped to my chest. I thought, *What? You want me to stick my husband with a needle? I'm not a nurse; I have great respect for nurses, but that doesn't mean I can be one!*

She smiled in understanding, but she didn't back off from her crazy idea. "You can do this," she encouraged. "You need to learn how to do this."

I nodded. "I know I've gotta learn how to do this, but what if I don't do it right? What if I hurt him? What if I kill him?" I tried to slow my breathing as I prayed for calmness.

As it so happened, we had a visitor at our house that day as well. I'll call him "Tim." He had been listening to our conversation and spoke up. "Evelyn, why don't you practice on me," he offered. "That way, you won't hurt Bob."

This conversation continued to surprise me. I thought, *I can't practice on this poor man. I'll hurt him.*

I shook my head. "I can't do that to you."

He insisted, and finally I gave in because they told me that Bob needed me to know how to do this. So, taking the needle in my hand, I followed the nurse's directions. Tim grimaced when I stuck him, and it pained me to know I hurt him.

"Try again," he said.

Oh, he sounded so brave. Reluctantly, I nodded and prayed some more. Then in my mind, I heard my mother's voice telling me that when she was sewing and had to thread the needle, she would always ask God to guide her hand, and He did. My sisters and I would chuckle because she couldn't see the hole at the head of the needle, yet she never missed threading it on the first try.

Then the calmness came. God would simply guide my hand too, just like he did my mother's.

I let out a deep breath and concentrated really hard. I placed the needle against Tim's arm, and God did it! He glided it in. It was easier than I thought!

When I went to give it to Bob, I was so nervous. I took his arm and touched him with the needle.

He yelled, "Ouch! Ouch! Ouch!"

Startled, I jumped back. I hadn't even put the needed in. He scared me so badly that I started crying.

"Oh honey, honey, don't cry," he pleaded in a soft and encouraging voice. "I was just trying to make you relax. I love you. You can do this."

I hesitated, and then I tried again, driven by the knowledge that my husband needed this so much. As it turned out, putting an IV in my husband's arm was easier than anticipated. I'm sure it hurt him, but he didn't show it. Instead, he immediately laid his head back.

"Oh my gosh!" he said, his voice now both excited and calm, "I can feel it, honey! I can feel it! It feels so good! I can feel it going up into my neck. It's amazing. Thank you so much! Thank you so much!"

I had no idea the IV could make such a difference for him. Pride and a sense of honor replaced my fear now that I knew I was able to give him so much immediate relief from his pain. Even though the fluids travelled all over his body, he would feel it go up into his throat area and lessen the tightness. It made him happy, and for that, I was thankful.

That night as I sat quietly by Bob, I thought of some of the Bible teachings concerning fear. I understood with greater clarity why "fear not" is stated so often in it. Fear not. How often would my sanity be saved by those two words?

Bob spoke, interrupting my thoughts. "It feels horrible when I can't get enough fluid to hydrate my body. That IV you gave me . . . you have no idea what you did for me."

Again, my heart burst with happiness. Seeing the impact of my efforts was the shot in the arm I needed to move forward in this battle for my husband's life.

−20−

A Child's Faith

The radiation unmercifully continued day after day. One afternoon while sitting in the waiting room of the radiation clinic, I noticed that Bob was having an exceptionally bad day. He was exhausted. The radiation was really taking a larger toll on him.

Looking back, I think we both probably looked a little beat around the edges. We didn't talk . . . just sat and stared straight ahead at nothing in particular and waited for someone to call his name for another treatment.

A woman sitting close by stood up and walked over to us. With a beautiful South African accent, she said, "Hello. My name is Liz Mews. Can I pray for you?"

"Yes, yes, please do," I eagerly accepted her invitation.

She looked back at the man who had been sitting next to her and nodded her head toward us. He got out of his chair and joined us.

"This is my husband, Aidan," she said, her smile warm. "Can he pray for you too?"

I nodded, blown away by the display of kindness and love shown by this couple. They both started praying for us. Afterward, we started talking with them.

"Are either of you going through radiation?" I asked.

Liz glanced at her husband and then looked at me. "No. Our son Motswedi has brain cancer. We actually live in London, but we came here for his treatments. His doctors there recommended this hospital as the best place to treat our son. We're waiting for him to finish his treatment." Her smile briefly faded and was replaced by the expression of a concerned mother.

Neither Aidan nor Liz looked old enough to have an adult child, so I asked, "How old's your son?"

"Eleven," Liz responded. "Eleven years old." Again, she inadvertently displayed a brief glimpse of a concerned mother. Then her smile returned. "But he's as strong as a lion," she proclaimed, "and he has such a strong faith in our Heavenly Father."

Impressed, I wanted to know as much about this couple and their son as possible. "Was he born in London?" I asked.

Then the grin of a proud mother emerged on Liz's face. "No. Motswedi—we call him 'Mots'—was born in Botswana, Southern Africa."

Ahh, now it made sense. "So that's the accent I'm hearing from you and your husband," I stated.

Liz nodded, and then her attention was diverted to a child entering the waiting room from the treatment area and walking to her. She held out her arms to welcome and envelop him in them.

She pulled back but kept her hands on the boy's shoulders. "This is our son Motswedi," she announced, that proud mama grin reappearing.

He turned to us with a huge smile on his face that belied the fact that he had just gone through another radiation treatment. "Hello," he said with a small wave.

His happy demeanor was contagious, inspiring, and gave me strength.

The Mews was a family I now wanted to be around. Just from that short time we spent in the waiting room together, their presence infused faith and peace inside me.

After Bob was called back for his treatment, I turned to the Mews and asked, "Why don't you come to our home for dinner?"

Liz and Aidan looked at each other before nodding.

Aidan answered, "Yes, we would like that very much."

From then on, it was like the Mews and the Kormondys were all going through this cancer treatment together. They came to our home frequently. While I would cook dinner, Liz, Mots, and I would dance in the family room. The men would laugh and enjoy our fun.

We took advantage of those times whenever we could because there were some days when no one felt like laughing. We just wanted to get through it, but somehow, we would get through it together. Their family was wrapped up in our family, and we were all wrapped up in God's love as one strong unit of faith.

As I spent more time with the Mews, I got to know more about Mots. His belief and faith in God were just as strong as the adults'. Although older than his years, he was still a child who loved going to the zoo because he loved lions. It wasn't hard to understand why. Lions were brave, and Mots was one of the bravest young men I had ever known with the kindest heart and biggest smile. He was also quite an artist. Of course, he loved to draw lions.

Months later when Bob started feeling better, I went back to work part time as a photographer for the Jacksonville Giants basketball team. Once I found out that Mots loved basketball, I told Joseph E. Miller, Vice President of Basketball Operations. He gave me tickets for Mots and his parents to attend the game with Bob and me. I was working the game, and Mots stayed on the floor with me, getting up-close views as I shot the pictures. It was a wonderful time. At the end, Joe also gave Mots a game T-shirt and some other wonderful memorabilia that meant so much to him.

By the grace of God, Mots ended up surviving brain cancer. We walked through that journey with him and his parents just like they walked through Bob's journey with us.

Undoubtedly, God had brought these friends to us during a time when we all needed it. We were there to encourage and support each other. He wanted us to see what they were going through as well as witness how strong they were despite their trials. We drew from their strength as we saw their faith to be something we all should strive to have.

The Mews became our forever friends. To this day, we still talk with them and celebrate milestones with them. This family blessed us more than they will ever know.

– 21 –

The Last Time

Thank God that the radiation treatments took place during the coldest months of the year, which in Florida were merely cool. The lower temperatures were a blessing because they made Bob's walks in and out of the clinic tolerable. We couldn't imagine his going through this burning experience and then having a hot Florida summer sun bearing down on him and scorching his skin even more while he walked to and from the car.

Still, the challenges persisted, even intensified. Despite all my efforts, Bob continued to lose weight because he wasn't getting enough Ensure. It broke my heart to constantly witness the changes in him, a man who was once full of life, strong, and could take on any wave with a surfboard. Now, his decline in that very strength and its consequential limitations prevented him from doing much of anything.

Since his surgery, he was only able to lift his arm shoulder-level. The skin had been pulled so tight that he could turn his head only so far.

Then toward the end of the radiation treatments, Bob got worse. He suffered from third-degree burns that required treatment using prescriptive creams and medicated bandages. He also became sensitive to sound, smell, and even touch. His weakness had gotten to the point that it was difficult for him to talk above a whisper, and I had to talk for him.

Of course, people wanted to help, to show him warmth, friendliness, and a good spirit, but Bob simply didn't have the strength. I became extremely adept at kindly blocking them from getting too close to him.

He told me I was his angel. That was one of the most wonderful things he had said to me because at that time, he needed an angel. I was glad it could be me.

It took everything he had in him to go through the motions of arriving at the radiation center, and I had to help him walk. Sitting in the waiting room gave him a little rest before they would call him to go back. He would force himself to walk down the hall, change, and get up onto the table so that they could strap his head to it with the mask and lie perfectly still so more radiation could be burned into his body and weaken it more. Afterward, he would climb off the table and manage to get himself dressed. This process happened time after time after time. The perpetual onslaught seemed as if it would never end.

Then he could barely walk back to the car, and I had to help him with that too. Our drives home were silent; he didn't even have the energy to talk. I understood and left him alone.

One night during that last week of radiation treatments, he managed to whisper, "When I'm in the room and strapped down by the mask, I feel like this isn't really happening to me, like this poor guy has to go through this horrible experience time and again. You know, I used to count all the radiation machine cycles, but now, all I can do is wait for the technicians to come in and take the mask off so that I can start living again. It seems like I die a little bit every time they strap on that mask."

His admission brought tears to my eyes. Although at the time, I didn't understand what going through massive doses of radiation was like, I did understand the repercussions. When he would come to me in the waiting room after undergoing a treatment, it about killed me to see how a little bit of life had left him back in that room.

Fortunately, Bob finally made it through those sixty-four radiation treatments in thirty-two excruciating days. He finally reached the light at the end of the tunnel at around 3:00 p.m. on Tuesday, March 1, 2012. Imagine the emotional high we felt, especially Bob, when the radiation came to an end!

Bob was Mercy Hospital's new radiation oncology clinic's first patient to ring the bell in the waiting room to signal he was done! He would never come back to the radiation room again!

Tears streamed down my face as I tried to process his joy as well as my own. Wow! What would our lives look like without this albatross around our necks!

After that sixty-fourth treatment, I helped Bob walk to the car, but he seemed lighter, almost as if he had a skip in his step. The world had somehow changed. The sun had boldly emerged from a long, cold, dark winter.

Before getting into our vehicle, we hugged and cried more before bowing our heads and thanking God for being with us every step of this devastating journey and bringing us through it . . . alive!

Yes, there would be checkups and other medical follow-ups in the future, but they were in the future. For now, nothing else mattered except this moment in time.

Joy and gratefulness filled our car as we headed east. With a huge smile on my face, I glanced over at Bob as he stared through the front window.

"Bob," I said, "take a look in the rearview mirror. Do you see it, Bob?"

"See what?" he whispered, a new strength resounding in his voice.

"The radiation clinic. Take one good last look at it in that mirror, Bob, because you're seeing that clinic for the last time!"

– 2 2 –

Life Without Radiation

Bob thrived in recovery mode. The surgery was done, chemotherapy was done, and radiation was done. Oh, how I love the word "done."

Still, things were difficult for Bob. When you've been at the bottom looking up, it can be a severely devasting place. The only hope you can grab onto comes from God as He gives you the comfort of knowing that nothing will be kicking you back down while you're working your way back up. And believe me, this was no small feat.

The radiation had created its own consequences, limitations, and relearning of what we all took for granted. Although Bob needed to learn how to turn his head, he couldn't start the therapy until he was healed from the third-degree burns caused by the radiation.

Then my sister Shirley stepped in. She was an amazing neuromuscular therapist and would come to the house to give Bob therapy. With her vast knowledge, she knew exactly what to do. Plus, he was very comfortable with her and appreciated her display of sensitivity over anyone touching his neck.

Shirley started giving him specialized myofascial therapy so that he could relearn how to move his jaw to chew. It was a process that would take a few months for him to get to the point that he could eat enough food to sustain his weight. Until then, the feeding tube would need to remain.

There were more challenges, too. One, Bob had fewer teeth to chew with as a result of the radiation, although he did get partial dentures to replace two. Another was the loss of his salivary glands. It not only gravely affected his taste buds and forced him to develop a new taste for food all over again, but it also affected his ability to swallow.

In Bob's case, however, it wasn't just relearning how to swallow again, but he had to eat in a way that would prevent him from choking. He would have to take tiny bites and dip them all into something with a liquid texture, such as gravies and ranch dressing (his favorite), to help his food go down.

Even with remastering his new skills of chewing and swallowing, there would be more learning and re-learning. For instance, he would have to drink water with every small bite. Also, he would need to be conscious of how much food he was consuming and could no longer rely on natural hunger to cue him when to eat.

He could no longer drink soft drinks (because they set his throat on fire) and wine (because of its dehydrating effects). The only options available to him were water and the next-best beverage—coffee! These changes were not temporary to get him through the healing process; they would become his new norm and a huge lifestyle change.

Nevertheless, Bob was eager to reclaim the rest of his life. From the day he got home from the hospital, he had one goal in mind—get back to work!

I did what I could, but Bob did his part; he was exceptionally motivated to get it done, get it done right, and get it done fast! The tightness and burn he had to suffer through had finally healed. He started the process to regain his ability to turn his head so that he would no longer need to turn his whole body from side to side to see something out of his peripheral vision.

Bob was breaking out of the confines he had been strapped into toward the end of the previous year.

It was 2012, and Bob was taking back his life!

– 2 3 –

Returning to His Passion

No sooner had Bob finished radiation than he went back to operating a television camera for NBC and CBS Sports as an independent contractor. Over the last two weeks, he had regained some strength and thought that if he didn't go back to work before long, he might not ever go back. His job had been his life, and he loved it! For a man as driven as Bob, there would have been no normal to his life without it.

Furthermore, there was the issue of money. Bob was anxious to start generating an income again. We hadn't been able to pay our bills for three months. Between all of the catching up we had to do and over $200,000 incurred in medical bills, we were now experiencing true financial hardship. So, we were thankful for the money!

His network directors were good to him, welcoming him back with open arms. That meant the world to

Bob. He knew he had a coveted position, but still, NBC Sports kept to their word that his job would be there for him when he was ready to go back. CBS Sports followed suit. Although their promise wasn't verbal, we knew they would be the same kind of wonderful company.

When Bob was ready, they wanted to make sure his transition to his new normal was rather easy, so they let him start off with a shortened workday. These thoughtful people were aware of Bob's limitations, which included the inability to raise his right arm above his shoulder. But to them, his eye and knowledge were more important.

To Bob, returning to work meant feeling useful again, and it allowed him to divert his attention away from what he had to endure daily. We will forever be grateful to the folks at NBC and CBS Sports for their kindness and help that allowed Bob to focus on restoring his life, finances, and health. We were far from out of the woods on any of those, but with each day, we got closer to the clearing.

Until then, Bob needed extra care at the end of his workday. He had to be given IVs, a shot of Vitamin B12, and much-needed nutrition through the feeding tube.

He also had ongoing appointments with Drs. Simpson, Davis, and Martin. Bloodwork was frequent, and he continued his neuromuscular therapy as well as other therapy to regain his range of motion in his neck.

Although Bob was all set to go back to work, he faced a challenge with his feeding tube. He refused to let it stop him, though; it was merely a challenge that he intended to overcome. So the medical staff had given us instructions on how to keep the tube sanitary and to deal with it in public when he was working. It wasn't going to be simple, and it required my presence with him wherever he was assigned to film.

Bob's first assignment was in Tampa to work a small golf tournament, which usually lasted about four hours. He especially enjoyed working these telecasts that aired live from his camera. He would have to make adaptations, though, such as the type of camera he used and his location for shooting.

His previous camera allowed him to walk the eighteen holes and cover the golfers. The problem was that it had to be carried on the right shoulder where Bob's surgery took place. Consequently, he was given a hard camera that he could place on a tripod in a fixed position and shoot from one location—on top of a covered camera tower.

Bob didn't have a problem operating the camera, but he would have to climb up and down the stairs with a feeding tube under his shirt. While on the tower, he would monitor when he would need water or Ensure. Then every hour, he would pour one of them into his feeding tube to make sure he stayed hydrated. During his lunch break, I would help.

So on March 14, 2012, I drove us to Tampa. The night before, I had packed him an extra suitcase full of IVs, bandages, medications, and Ensure. The first few days consisted of meetings and preparations, and then on March 17, he shot his first sporting event in four months.

He was like a kid, full of excitement and eagerness despite the adjustments in how he performed his job. He didn't care. He was back in his world, doing what he did best. He was the ultimate professional, determined to work around the inconveniences.

Then every night in the hotel room, I administered his treatments (IVs, medication, and wound care) as well as poured the proper nourishment into his feeding tube again. They were all essential to get him through the next day.

We left from Tampa on March 18 and spent the next three days recuperating before driving to the beautiful Arnold Palmer's Bay Hill Club & Lodge in Orlando, Florida, on March 21. As with Tampa, Bob would shoot the golf tournament during the day, and then at night, we were alone again with Ensure, medications, IV bags, and medical equipment.

Some thought that we had a sad life, but we never considered ourselves as anything but blessed. Bob had survived cancer . . . twice . . . and we were living the life. I hadn't seen that glean in his eyes in quite some time. He was doing what he loved.

I was getting my husband back, something I didn't take for granted. I would have gone to the ends of the earth with him with Ensure in tow, to make sure he had the nutrition and energy he needed and just to be near him.

And then we had to head back to Jacksonville where bloodwork and doctor appointments beckoned him, distracting him from his passion. However, he couldn't afford to neglect them. After all, doing what they told him to do was the crux of why he was still alive.

So on March 27, Bob had a full day of bloodwork and appointments with Drs. Martin and Simpson, and then the next day, with Dr. Davis. He soon learned that spending two hours in a doctor's office was much more exhausting than two hours up on the tower.

−24−

Imminent Foreclosure

As I relished in Bob's progress and how proud I was of him, I got hit with news that took my breath away.

Ever since our mortgage lender had offered us a hardship refinance with our mortgage, I had been calling them every week. And every week, they affirmed that the refi process was going along fine. Now that the three-month grace period was almost up, I called again to check the status. Plus, I needed to make our May payment.

I spoke to the same representative. She didn't merely assure me all was fine, but she told me that the refi was almost done. Feeling encouraged, I carried on with my activities.

Imagine my surprise when later that day, someone unexpectedly rang our doorbell. Upon opening it, a middle-aged man holding a clipboard smiled as he asked. "Evelyn Kormondy?"

"Yes. I'm Evelyn Kormondy," I responded somewhat perplexed. *Do I know you?* I wondered.

He pulled some papers from his clipboard and handed them to me. "You've been served."

"Served with what?" I asked, completely confused.

I glanced down at what he had just handed me. *Foreclosure papers?*

"What?" I asked, not able to understand. "This can't be from our mortgage company. Why would they serve me with foreclosure papers? Our house is getting refinanced. I just got through talking with them today, and they confirmed that it was almost done. The representative at the bank told me that they were still working on it, and it looked like it was going to be accepted because of our great credit history with them."

The stranger shrugged his shoulders and then turned and walked away.

I stood immobilized for a few moments before I was able to force myself to go inside. After closing the door behind me, I put my head against it and cried as silently as I could. Bob didn't need to hear me, and he didn't need to know what was happening. He needed to heal. This was a mistake, and I needed to call our mortgage lender and get it all cleared up.

I went into a room far away from Bob and called the bank on my cell phone. The same representative answered.

"Hi. This is Evelyn Kormondy," I began, forcing myself to remain calm and steady. "I just got served with foreclosure papers from our mortgage company. It says they're foreclosing on our home on September 13."

"Yes, ma'am. It looks like that way," she responded with absolutely no emotion in her voice.

I was more than shocked. Obviously, I needed to show her the absurdity of the situation and remind her of our conversations. "But you told me everything was fine," I argued, "that the refi was almost done. I even have it writing."

You will not hear me cry, I screamed in my head.

The representative had obviously taken on a different tone than she had in any of our calls in the past, and it didn't appear that she was warming up to me and empathizing with our dilemma one bit. "It doesn't matter, Mrs. Kormondy. You're delinquent in your mortgage payments, so we're going to need to foreclose on your home."

"I didn't make mortgage payments because you told me not to make mortgage payments, that it would mess up the refinance process. Every week when I called, you kept telling me that the refi was almost done. In fact, just a few hours ago, you told me it looked like it was going to be accepted!"

"Well, it's not. They're not refinancing your home, Mrs. Kormondy. We're taking it back. It's been three months since you've made a payment."

This couldn't possibly be happening. She sounded firm with a take-it-or-leave-it attitude and that there was no room for arguments or negotiations.

"How much do we need to pay to keep it out of foreclosure?" Tears ran down my cheeks.

"Uhm . . . let me see. With interest and late payment fees, ten thousand dollars." I've heard more emotion from people sharing the weather.

I wiped the tears from my cheeks with the back of my hand. "Ten thousand dollars? But I don't have ten thousand dollars. You know our situation. You know what my husband's been through. I've sent you all of the paperwork you've asked for to verify our financial predicament. My husband's in the next room, for heaven's sake, with IVs in his arm." I pleaded, trying again to get her to see the logic since trying to touch upon her sense of humanity didn't seem to be an option.

"Then you'll just have to put him in a wheelchair and get out," she retorted, sounding almost menacing.

What a mean thing to say! I hung up and broke down. We've been through so much, and now we were losing our home? It didn't make any sense. I had done everything our mortgage lender told me to do, and now, they were using my following their directions against us.

I had no choice at this time; I had to tell Bob what was happening. He would want to know; he needed to know. He was such a good man, always making sure he took care of me, and together, we knew God was taking care of both of us. But now that I was supposed to take care of him, well, we can see how that was working out.

After composing myself the best I could, I walked into the family room and sat on the couch next to Bob. He eyed me with both concern and curiosity.

"Evie, what's wrong? Who was at the door?" he asked.

I let out a big sigh and broke down again. I tried so hard to be brave, to do this on my own, but I was failing miserably at both.

Once I calmed down enough to speak, I stated, "Bob, that was a process server."

His eyebrows furrowed in complete confusion. "Process server?" he repeated. "Why would a process server be knocking at our door?"

I squeezed my eyes shut momentarily as I tried to come up with the right words, but there were no right words. He just needed to hear about what was going on, and at this point, there was no way to sugar coat it.

"He was here to serve us with foreclosure papers from our mortgage company." I could barely look at him.

Bob didn't say anything, probably because he was trying to make sense out of the news I had just dumped on him. "I don't understand," he finally responded, his words slow and full of uncertainty.

I proceeded to tell him the story, about everything that had transpired since January with our mortgage lender and our mortgage. I told him about my weekly follow-up calls to the representative, her weekly assurances that all was well, and her warnings to not make a payment because it would confuse the refinance process.

It was hard going through the sequence of events without lamenting along the way. Bob's eyes went from bewilderment of what was happening to anger over what the bank had done to us and to me, and then to compassion for me.

He wrapped his left arm around my shoulder and kissed the top of my head. "Evie, I am so sorry you went through this on your own. You didn't need to do this all by yourself. You have already taken on way too much. From now on, please let me know these kinds of things. I'm a big boy; I can take it. My body may be healing, but my mind works just as good as it always has."

Oh, how I loved this man!

"That's okay," I responded. "I'm here for you; that's where I'm supposed to be. Your only job is to get better."

He wiped my tears from my face. "I worry about you, Evie."

"Don't," I responded. "This is my job right now—to protect you. It's my turn to be strong for you because you've always been the strong one. You have more strength than anybody I know to endure what you're going through. Right now, it's taking everything you have just to get through each day. God and me, we've got this."

My words sounded brave, but inside, I was crumbling.

Bob must have sensed my forced façade. "Let's just go ahead and pray about this together."

We did. When sickness, pain, and injustice came against us, this was how we fought back . . . on our knees. And during those times when we were physically unable to get on our knees, we just held each other and put our requests before God.

Over the next week, I shared what had happened with some friends and people at church. At this point, we needed prayers. Our mortgage lender seemed determined to take our home away from us, and only God could help.

A couple of weeks later after the church service, some of our friends approached me. "Evelyn, is it okay if we come over to your house this afternoon? It's important."

"Sure," I answered. This was strange, and I was curious as to what they wanted.

I went home and told Bob that some of the people from church wanted to come by. We both assumed it was to see him. Soon afterward, they started arriving at our home. I invited them all inside.

Some of them went into the family room to talk to Bob, but the others were removing photography pictures from my walls. I had shot all of them, blown them up, and framed them to help decorate the rooms.

Confused, I asked, "What are you doing?"

They all looked at me and smiled. "We're buying your pictures from you, Evelyn. And we're paying you double."

"No, no. You don't have to do that. Plus, if I sold them to you, I'd charge you less anyway."

"Evelyn, we wanna help. We know we can't just give you money; you won't take it. So we all decided to buy your photography. That way, you'll have the satisfaction of earning the money."

My eyes pooled with tears and fell unashamedly down my face. By the time the "sale" was over, I had more than ten thousand dollars. We could now pay our mortgage lender and get our home out of foreclosure.

Our problem was now resolved! I almost ran into the family room to share the news with Bob! He had been so preoccupied with talking to whomever was in the room with him that he no idea what was occurring in the other rooms.

"Look how this whole situation ended up, how God came through and provided!" I exclaimed. "We're a team—you, God, and me!"

We then praised God for His goodness and faithfulness.

It was obvious I wasn't in this battle alone. Where I was weak, God proved Himself strong. He knew I needed His strength now more than ever.

God had heard our cries, and He had heard our prayers. In response, He had sent His angels in the forms of wonderful friends to meet our needs.

– 2 5 –

No More Feeding Tube!

And then Bob was assigned to work the Master's Tournament in Augusta, Georgia from April 3 to April 8. It was a big deal because it was one of the largest golf tournaments of the year. Consequently, it would require him to work longer days. By then, however, he was able to do whatever it took!

He soared through the Master's Tournament. Obviously, he was gaining strength, which was needed because for the month of May 2012, our life was one golf tournament after another. First it was the TPC (The Players Championship) in Jacksonville, Florida from May 8–13, and then two days later, the Nationwide Tour in Greenville, South Carolina from May 15–21, and the next day, the PGA Senior Championship in Indiana. Our month was a whirlwind of travel, work, and nighttime IVs in hotel rooms.

Tired, we would come home from all these exciting places at the end of the month and have to pivot back to our other life, the one where Bob was under close medical supervision for the nightmare we just woke up from. So he would have to go back to see his doctors on a monthly basis for follow-ups and blood work.

Although these office visits wore us both out, Bob got a metaphorical shot in the arm. On June 2, less than six months after undergoing a radical neck dissection, he miraculously played golf for the first time since Australia with his surgeon, Dr. Simpson, at the Amelia River Golf Club. Because Dr. Simpson would know better than anyone what Bob could and couldn't do as a result of the surgery, Bob felt comfortable playing with him.

But during their game, Bob became devasted when he realized he didn't have the same swing as he did prior to his surgery. He had been an extremely good golfer, but his limitation with his right arm changed his game. He used to hit a perfect draw with a solid divot. Now, he had lost twenty-five yards of distance on all his irons. Although understandably disappointed, he figured out how he would adapt his game to fit his new normal, and Dr. Simpson was quite impressed.

In addition to his limitations, he was doing all this with a feeding tube. For Bob, he confronted every obstacle head-on. Each challenge would learn that it adapted to Bob's life, not the other way around.

Having your surgeon play golf you with was quite a blessing. Dr. Simpson was great at explaining the whys of Bob's limitations. But one cannot discount the wisdom shared by those without medical degrees or certificates, those who had acquired knowledge and perspective from actually going through the same thing, those who could tell you about how they fared, even survived it firsthand.

For Bob, that person had been Jason, a friend of our neighbor Kevin. Back when Kevin found out that Bob was getting a feeding tube, he told him about Jason because he had managed a restaurant while wearing a feeding tube. As a result, he had learned how to address the challenges and needs involved.

Bob appreciated the opportunity to talk to someone else who had been there, done that, and as a result, could offer tried-and-proven solutions on how to survive it all. He called Jason, and they talked for over an hour. Based on his own experiences, he told Bob what to expect from the feeding tube.

Jason was honest as he prepared Bob for the good, the bad, and the ugly so that he would not be surprised at natural occurrences, such as the feeding tube adjustments that would need to be done at certain times during the day. And by the way, they would not be convenient, especially at work.

Bob listened tentatively to Jason's stories, such as how he would have to take a break at work and lie down on the restaurant's bar and have somebody help adjust his feeding tube. Afterward, he was able to resume his responsibilities.

If Jason could do it while working an active job, then so could Bob. Sure, he would have to stop everything momentarily for an adjustment that would surely demand his attention, but it was all doable.

In the end, Jason taught Bob more than how to manage a feeding tube at a physical job; Jason helped Bob get through a very difficult time and demonstrated how imperative it was to have someone counsel you through traumatic events. Bob was given hope that in spite of having a feeding tube, he could recapture an important part of his life.

And he did! Those conversations came back in full force when we were confronted with the issues Jason had prewarned Bob about earlier. And boy, did we appreciate the advice! Thanks to Jason, we were able to successfully work through those inconveniences.

We found comfort as well as motivation in knowing that his feeding tube was temporary, and soon, this too shall end when the doctor took it out for good. But when that would take place would be up to Bob and how he progressed.

Again, Bob's a fighter and a determined one at that. He may get knocked down, but watch out! He forces himself back onto his feet and starts punching back.

Over the months, Bob had been punching back by working hard in and between his therapy appointments, and it paid off. That June when we were in Dr. Martin's office, Bob was able to inform him that he could now swallow and was doing better overall.

Evidently, the report was good enough for Dr. Martin to schedule the removal of Bob's feeding tube for the following week. So after four long months of

Ensure, Bob was going to regain even more of his life and independence. It was a giant leap forward.

Excitement couldn't help but be built up in those days approaching the procedure. Removing the tube wasn't as big of a deal as inserting it, so I could be with him when they took it out.

When the removal date came, Bob and I arrived at the outpatient surgical center at Mercy. We were like two kids eagerly anticipating Christmas morning.

After checking in and a nurse getting Bob's vitals, we were led to one of their surgical rooms. Bob was told to get up on the table and lie back.

Dr. Martin came into the room. "Let's get this tube out of you now, Bob," he announced with a grin.

The doctor allowed me to stand next to Bob and hold his hand. By this point in our journey, nothing bothered me. Although we were told what would happen during the procedure, I was quite curious to see it in real time.

Dr. Martin said, "Okay, Bob, take a deep breath."

He did, and voila! The doctor easily and smoothly pulled out the tube with the ball attached at the end.

Now that it was gone, the hole in Bob's stomach sucked itself closed right there in front of us. It was an interesting phenomenon and an amazing sight!

After monitoring the event a few moments more, the doctor said, "You need to lie on the table for about an hour to give it time to finish closing naturally." He then left the room, and a nurse took over.

Once the hour was over, she glanced up at the black and white clock hanging on the white wall. She announced, "Well, it's been an hour. Looks like you can leave."

Bob sat up and got off the table. "It feels great to have that thing finally out!" he exclaimed.

We left the room, and Bob went to get dressed. We walked about halfway to the waiting area when a small amount of clear liquid started coming out of the hole in his stomach, spilling onto his shirt and the floor. He looked down and then at me. I stood frozen in shock as I tried to process what had just happened and what to do about it.

Once I came to my senses, I yelled out, "Excuse me. We have a problem. Somebody? Hello?"

Two nurses rushed over to us. The older one remarked, "Oh, it's okay. We just need you to come back in and lie back down on the table a little longer."

They helped Bob walk back to the room and onto the table. Now that the initial shock was over, Bob and I started laughing, some out of relief once we realized it wasn't a big deal, but mostly because it seemed funny at the time.

I jested, "Goodness gracious, honey. Can't keep things in your stomach."

After about another thirty minutes of lying still on the table, I guessed the hole finally did what it was supposed to do—close completely. Of course, it looked completely closed the first time too. Regardless, we took our chances and left, and Bob never had another problem with it again.

Bob told Jason after the feeding tube was removed. Over the months of radiation and having a feeding tube, the two men had developed a camaraderie. He asked Bob, our daughters, and me to come to his restaurant and have dinner with him. It would be Bob's first meal out in a restaurant since his surgery and without a feeding tube in his stomach.

Jason brought out a bottle of wine for us to share, but Bob didn't even touch it. Instead, Bob ordered water for his drink and a light meal with shrimp. I ordered a fillet steak.

Although Bob didn't eat much, his perpetual smile and relaxed demeanor showed that he was happy. Afterward, he told me that it felt good to be in the presence of somebody who knew what he was going through at that moment and that dinner was the highlight of his relationship with Jason, one he would never forget.

To this day, they are still friends.

−26−

Defying the Odds

By the end of June and all of July, Bob's schedule continued to be packed with one golf tournament after the other. We travelled from city to city, and in each one, we had to stay between three days and a whole week. The most memorable was again the annual American Century Celebrity Golf Championship Tournament in Lake Tahoe that Bob worked every year for NBC Sports. In 2012, it took place from July 17 to July 22.

Since Bob no longer had a feeding tube, I didn't need to be with him while he worked. So I was able to shoot the tournament as a photographer for a magazine. While I was on the ground taking pictures, Bob was up on his camera tower. We were back working together again, and it felt great!

I recognized Oscar De La Hoya, the professional boxer and promoter. He had a crowd of spectators around him, and he was signing autographs. That evening, I went to a local sporting goods store and bought a pair of boxing gloves.

The next day when I saw Oscar at the tournament, I approached him and held up the gloves. "Mr. De La Hoya, I'm Evelyn Kormondy, and I'm here shooting pictures for a magazine."

He smiled as he stared at the gloves.

"Would you mind autographing these?" I asked.

A slow smile spread across his face as his eyes showed understanding, and he nodded. What a kind man! As his pen glided across the gloves with his signature, I told him about Bob, that he was a camera operator on hole 15, that he was my husband, a fan, and what he had gone through. Bob had no idea I had even met Oscar, let alone talked to him.

Oscar signed the boxing gloves "Keep fighting, Bob!" Then when he got to hole 15, he pointed to Bob's camera and made an uppercut punch to encourage him to keep up the fight. Then he shouted, "Bob Kormondy!"

Of course, Bob wasn't quite sure what was happening, but he waved back at Oscar anyway. When I saw Bob later on, I explained that I had met Oscar De La Hoya and told him about his cancer.

He smiled, looking pleased. "Oh, that was why he did what he did."

During that same event, I had another encounter with a celebrity—eleven-time world surfing champion Kelly Slater who also played in this golf tournament. Bob had already met Kelly several times beforehand because they had a few things in common. First, they were both surfers. Second, Kelly is from Cocoa Beach, Florida, and Bob grew up a few minutes away in Satellite Beach.

During one of his breaks, I approached Kelly and said, "Hi, Kelly." I then let him know that Bob was back working the tournament after fighting cancer and was stationed on hole 15

He listened intently before sharing with me how his father had died of throat cancer. It was the same kind of cancer that Bob had. Kelly then told me about a great recipe that Bob should be drinking every day. Even though he had to get back to the course soon, he took the time to write that recipe on a piece of paper for Bob.

He instructed me, "Make sure he drinks this every day."

Bob did and still does.

That tournament turned out to be the turning point where Bob felt like he was truly getting his life back. Having the feeding tube removed was important physically, but the support, encouragement, and recognition from family and friends were crucial. He was fortunate to have three people he admired, world champions who recognized the struggle he was going through—a windsurfer who had mailed him a windsurfing board, a boxer who recognized him during a tournament, and a surfer who gave him a drink recipe for his health and healing.

And then . . . back to the medical world of monthly doctor visits with some lab work sprinkled throughout. Thankfully, all was well. We left these appointments feeling like we were stepping back into our other dimension where our lives and passions were thriving and flourishing. The doctors recognized Bob's need to work. They approved his hectic schedule and allowed him to arrange his appointments with them around his sporting events.

In addition, Bob started reengaging more and more in the sports activities he had once enjoyed. Sure, he had some ground to make up, but with each one, he was disproving Dr. Martin's prophecy that he would never play sports again. Ha! He did not know my Bob! He shocked Dr. Martin when he showed him a video of him surfing. But it was a good shock because he was so proud of Bob!

And he should be because surfing had been a challenge. When Bob first tried after the cancer treatments, he couldn't lift his arm high enough to clear the water while paddling to catch a wave. Afterwards, while we were in a surf shop, he came across a special vest he could wear that would raise his chest an inch off the surfboard, just enough to let his arm clear the water. He then eventually began standup paddleboarding to get his exercise in the water.

With his determination, he displayed his relentlessness to defy the odds, not just with surfing but with other sports as well, such as golf. Fortunately, his brother was a golf pro and helped him with his swing. Bob would also tee the golf ball up the fairway so that he could make solid contact with the ball. Otherwise, if the club hit the ground with any force, he would get an instant shock to the base of his skull, which caused him to get a headache. With every game, he continued taking the good with the bad and adapt more to a new way to play golf.

Since then, Bob created a golf swing. He used to hit a draw, and now he hits a fade. He plays a closer tee box for shorter distance, and he's able to hit more fairways and more greens in regulation. The distances of each of his irons are very exact, and he's not able to overswing his club.

Before the surgery, Bob played with a six handicap. Afterwards, he had a round of golf where he hit every fairway off the tee and every green in regulation for an even-par round. He had thought this would be impossible after the surgery, but it became possible because of his adaptions.

He then took his perseverance to another passion—archery. Whereas before the surgery, he shot right-handed with a thirty-inch draw. Post-surgery, he could only pull twenty-five inches. What did he do? Adapt! After all, he had always been able to help others reach their goals of a consistent grouping with a recurve bow, and now it was time for the teacher to teach himself. That involved relearning how to shoot left-handed. He had seen others online shooting with both hands, so he figured, "Why not me? Why not give it a try?"

Not surprisingly, he achieved success and currently has a perfect draw of thirty inches with his left hand. In fact, he believes he shoots better with his left hand than he does with his right. If not for the surgery, he would have never taught himself to shoot with his other hand.

His main sporting passion, though, was windsurfing. Using his new windsurfing board that Francisco Goya gave him, it wasn't long before he was once again able to windsurf in winds of up to forty miles per hour, a feat that's difficult to accomplish, even for someone who hasn't undergone surgery or radiation. But Bob achieved it with confidence.

Fortunately, most of the control of the sail is done in front of the body, and he has normal movement there and is able to control the sail with normal action. His only challenge would be swimming back to the board if he fell and got separated from it. He has to swim on his side with one arm.

He tried all the others sports he used to play, such as ice skating and ice hockey. He had to adapt to less energy and the way he handled his stick and took a wrist shot. Then when he was able to compete, he felt a real sense of accomplishment.

Admittedly, he could find himself frustrated when he couldn't perform these activities like he used to, but he always took it as a challenge to figure out a way to adapt.

His positive refuse-to-give-up attitude overflowed into everything he got involved with. As a result, life went on as together, we adjusted to a new normal.

The holidays came and went in 2012, but for Christmas, Bob was able to resume helping with the decorations. However, the major difference between this Christmas and the previous one could be felt in the atmosphere—joy and gratitude had replaced apprehension and fear.

Bob was definitely back, back to traditional family activities and back to work, leaving home for periods at a time to shoot a sporting event in another city, another state, another country.

Before we knew it, time was also flying through 2013. All was well.

Until it wasn't.

$-27-$

Was That a Lump

It began just like any other Saturday but ended unlike any other Saturday I've ever experienced. It's date—June 15, 2013—will be forever etched in my mind.

Bob was covering the 16 green of the U.S. Open near Philadelphia, and I was at home watching it on TV. The afternoon sun streamed through the window, and I enjoyed its warmth caressing the side of my face.

Then the tournament went to commercial. As I turned to glance out the window, I scratched the side of my left breast and froze.

What just happened? Was that a lump?

Fear overcame me, heat rose within me, and I couldn't breathe. Although I had never had breast cancer myself, it wasn't a stranger to me. I knew what a lump meant, and I knew I was at high risk of getting it. One of my sisters had died from breast cancer, and another one was a survivor of it.

I had a sick feeling in my stomach that I was in deep, deep trouble. I started crying.

The U.S. Open came back on TV, but I couldn't see it through the blur created by my tears. It was the weekend, and my doctor's office was closed. Although an emergency to me, he couldn't do anything about it today. I would have to wait until Monday, the same day Bob was coming home from the U.S. Open. He had already gone through so much, so I didn't want to tell him anything until I knew for sure.

Still, in my heart, I knew . . . I just knew.

An ominous feeling started to develop and hover in the atmosphere, so I got up to take a shower in the hopes that it would make me feel better. I plodded to my bathroom, each of my legs seemingly weighing at least 500 pounds.

As the water ran over me, I hesitantly felt for that same lump. Maybe I had been sitting at a bad angle, and I had mistaken something quite innocent for it. Holding my breath with great hope and optimism, I felt the side of my left breast again, and there it was, definitely a lump that didn't belong there.

I lay in bed that night thinking about my sister

Scottie who didn't survive breast cancer and all that she went through—the pain, the surgery, the chemo. It was just too much for her, and the cancer spread throughout her body.

Then I thought about everything my sister Maria had gone through with her breast cancer. What did she do differently to survive it?

Of course, I thought about Bob. Although he hadn't gone through breast cancer, his cancer was vicious, and in return, he had to fight back even more viciously.

What would I say to him if I'm told the lump is cancer? Undoubtedly, the news would devastate him.

Finally, sleep overcame my weary mind, but the fear of cancer merely followed me into my dreams, stalking me unmercifully. I dreamt that it had already spread throughout my body. It seemed so real and scared me so much that I woke up crying. I felt like I had a fever but realized my temperature had probably increased due to the anxiety and what it was putting my body through. I was overwhelmed with questions as to what to do and wondering if I was going to die or survive.

Monday was so far away. Breathing once again became difficult, so I got up and went into the family room. It was more open than my bedroom and didn't seem to close in on me.

Exhausted yet unable to sleep, I sat on the couch. I thought, *At some point, surely, I'll fall asleep, and when I do, it could be right here in this open room.*

Turned out, I didn't sleep at all. Instead, I sat on that couch all weekend focused on what Monday was going to bring. Then I would remind myself about God's supernatural power. Why would he bring Bob through cancer only to let me die? It didn't make sense.

So I prayed, and I prayed. But deep down, I knew I had cancer.

The next morning, I went to our Sunday church service, but I didn't tell anyone about the lump. I stayed afterward and went into our church's small chapel alone and silently prayed to my Heavenly Father to guide me and to give me the strength I needed. Only He could bring me through it. Afterward, I went home and prayed more. It was the only thing I could do at that point.

Finally, Monday morning arrived. I got out of bed at six after another night with no sleep. Instead, I had watched the hands of the clock slowly move with the sound of a steady and monotonous tick tock, tick tock, tick tock in the background.

Just two and a half hours to go, two and a half hours of waiting, waiting, waiting for the hour hand to make its way to the eight on the clock and the minute hand to the five.

In the meantime, I fixed a cup of coffee and got dressed, all the while keeping an eye on the clock, willing its hands to move faster. My gynecologist's office would not open until 8:30, but at 8:25, I gripped my phone tightly and stood in position with my finger on the keyboard buttons, ready to dial the second they opened their phone lines.

Finally, 8:30!

After punching in the memorized number, I held my breath as their phone rang. Standing still was almost impossible.

Thankfully, someone answered on the third ring. "Dr. Michael Smith's office."

I explained what I had found. "Please, can I see the doctor today?" I begged. By now, I was about to jump out of my skin while waiting to hear her answer.

"Yes, Evelyn. Come in right away."

Whew!

I hung up the phone. Dr. Smith's office wasn't very far away, and I had already put everything I would need in place so that when it was time to go, I could just grab it and leave.

With blinders on, I rushed to my car and started the drive so that I could finally find out what that lump was about. At least the day was beautiful, which helped my mood somewhat. I turned on my car radio and sang along to the songs in an effort to get my mind off of what was to come.

Then the beautiful day became blurred and the music muffled as a barrage of questions took over my thoughts. *How can I be sick?* I wondered, finding ludicrousness in this whole crazy idea that I could have cancer. *I feel so good. How can anything be wrong with me? I'm so happy. Bob had survived. How could I be sick? This can't be happening. This just can't be happening.*

Once I arrived at Dr. Smith's office, I signed in. The nurse looked up from her desk. "We'll be right with you, Evelyn."

I found a seat in the waiting room. Minutes seemed like hours.

How long is it going to take to know something? Please, somebody, let me know something, I silently pleaded, forcing myself not to scream my thoughts out loud.

After being called back to the cold room, I got undressed and sat on the padded exam table. Then more rationalizing and minimizing: *Maybe he won't examine me. If he doesn't, then that proves he doesn't think anything's wrong. After all, it could just be my imagination. I'm making too much out of nothing. That's it. I shouldn't be here.*

Dr. Smith came in fairly quickly. His warm and kind demeanor usually calmed me down, but not today. I was too wound up.

"Maybe everything's okay, Evelyn, but I'll take a look," he stated optimistically.

Okay, I'll go with that, I thought. *Maybe everything's okay.*

I nodded and lay back holding my left arm over my head while turning my head to the right. Dr. Smith's hand was cold, the room was cold, my life was cold. Everything was cold.

He examined me and then examined me again.

"Okay, Evelyn. Go ahead and get dressed. Then come meet me in my office." He turned to leave.

That's it? He's not going to say anything? He's just going to leave and make me wait more?

Before he could go, I asked, "Dr. Smith, are things not okay?"

He turned back to me with a smile. "I'll meet you in my office."

Wow! Now I was really scared. This was not my first rodeo. I've been through this meet-you-in-my-office directive with Bob's doctors. By now, I kind of knew the playbook.

I got dressed as quickly as I could and then trudged down the hall to his office. It was empty. I sat down in one of the chairs in front of his desk and waited for what seemed like forever. I tried to occupy my mind with something else by looking at the pictures of his wife and family. They only made me think of my own family, which made me think about my circumstances.

What am I going to do? What's going to happen to my family? What's going to happen to my husband? I don't understand.

Finally, Dr. Smith came into the office and sat down behind his desk. "Evelyn, you have a lump. It's solid and we've gotta go see what it's all about. You need to go to the Cox Breast Clinic near Crestview Hospital downtown. I've made an appointment, and you need to go right away."

I wanted to argue that this was silly, a waste of everyone's time. Instead, I asked, "When's the appointment?"

"Wednesday. Day after tomorrow."

His definition and my definition of "right away" were obviously way off. Wednesday felt like a hundred years away. It was only Monday and Monday morning at that.

Why can't they see me now? Why can't I find out right now what is happening?

My head spun. It was all too much to process.

Dr. Smith walked me down the hall with his arm around my shoulders. "You'll be in the best of hands, Evelyn. They'll take really good care of you," he stated in a calm, reassuring voice.

But there was no reassuring me. My life had just been through a horrible, horrible time with Bob. I reflected on all the appointments, all the concerns I had about his medications, so worried that I wouldn't give him what he needed at the right time.

The memories created so much stress that I couldn't breathe. I walked out to the car, climbed in, and closed the door. Then I sobbed and sobbed and sobbed for I don't know how long.

During the drive home, I thought about Bob. In a few hours, he would be home for a couple of days. There was no way I could tell him tonight, not until I knew for sure. I couldn't worry him like this.

I took a shower as soon as I got home, thinking that maybe I could wash away the day. Maybe if I took a long enough shower, I would wake up from this nightmare.

I played some music from my playlist on my phone and tried to pump myself up. Afterward, I got all pretty for my husband because I loved him so much. Then I waited for him to walk through our front door, trying not to cry, reminding myself that crying would ruin my makeup.

How was I going to keep this from him until I knew for sure? How could I keep my face from showing I had this scary secret?

Dear Lord, please give me strength.

−28−

Keeping Secrets

The sound of our front door closing signaled that the taxi had just dropped Bob off from the airport. He was now home with me for a little while before he would have to pack up and leave again.

I stopped straightening up our bedroom and walked out to greet him.

He walked over to me with a big smile on his face, obviously happy to see me. He looked so handsome, so strong.

The big smile on my face wasn't forced because I was so happy to see him too. He was great medicine for me right now.

We gave each other a kiss and a big hug. Then reality slapped me across the face, cruelly reminding me of the lump. It was all I could do to act as if everything was fine, to not show the terror I felt about the probable cancer growing slowly in my body.

When he pulled back, he paused and studied my face. "Evie," he said with compassion, "sweetheart, there's a tear in your eye."

I guess I didn't try hard enough. "I'm crying because I'm so happy to see you," I responded. It was true, well, that and because of the panic. "I'm so glad you're home. I've missed you so much. How was your trip?" I wanted to distract his focus off me.

It worked. He talked about his trip while putting away his bags, and I listened as attentively as possible. In the back of my mind, though, I kept hearing, *You've got cancer, Evelyn. Cancer. Cancer. Cancer.*

We then put on some music, and I fixed dinner. Bob grabbed me from behind and twirled me around to dance with him in the kitchen. It was like the old days when everything was so beautiful. The surroundings, the music, the laughter, dancing—everything seemed to be okay.

Maybe I wasn't sick after all. Maybe I just thought I was. Yes, I was going to go with that for now. It was the only option I had to keep me from thinking about the doom so that I could simply be happy being with Bob in the moment.

That evening, I lay in Bob's arms like I had a thousand times before. It was my favorite place to fall asleep.

I silently prayed, *Thank You, God, for Bob and for his survival. We know that You, Heavenly Father, will help us through this, whatever it is. We know that You will give us strength.*

I fell asleep, still in Bob's arms, with the reassurance that God was with me.

When I woke up the next morning, it felt good to have Bob next to me. I snuggled in his arms and pondered all that laid ahead. And I still didn't know if something was wrong with me; that answer wouldn't come until tomorrow when I went to Cox Breast Clinic. The tortuous unknown began once again consuming my thoughts.

Despite my anxiety, I had to go through my normal routine so that I could appear normal. Fortunately, I could do it all with my eyes shut—make coffee, make breakfast, ask Bob how he's feeling, give him his medications, check for his appointments, check for his follow-ups, unpack his suitcase, do laundry, everything that I had always done for him when he came home from a trip. In the midst of these tasks, we would do fun things together. It would be good for me.

So, I smiled and laughed on the outside, but on the inside, I was going nuts and was terrified. I hated having to keep this major secret from my best friend, the one person I trusted most in life, and my confidante.

I put myself on autopilot and went through my routine step-by-step, going above and beyond, thinking of what I needed to do in case something horrible happened to me, doing a mental checklist as I smiled at Bob and cooked his breakfast.

In spite of the bad, I was able to have fun and be the second half of Evie and Bob. We played as much as we could and did what needed to be done, all with the knowledge that God was with us; He had been with us the whole time.

I resolved myself to praise Him today, enjoy today, love today, and laugh today. That was all I could do for now, although by the end of that day, I was exhausted. However, I was proud that I had handled it by myself.

I thought, *I can do this.*

No sooner had my confidence built than it started to fall when that baleful voice at the back of my mind asked, *But what about tomorrow? I have to go to the breast center alone. Am I going to be able to handle that by myself? What if the news is bad? How am I going to handle that? What about Bob? How would I tell him? No, no, I can't tell him until the absolute last minute. I need to wait until I know for sure. When will I know for sure?*

Please, somebody, stop the screaming inside my head! Stop the screaming inside my head!

I found myself actually smiling and screaming inside my head simultaneously!

By the time we crawled into bed that night, Bob didn't suspect anything. He had no idea cancer could be spreading inside my body just like it had spread inside his.

The next day, I woke up early before him and made coffee. While it brewed, I read my morning devotionals and prayed. Today was *the* day—Wednesday, June 19, Cox Breast Clinic where someone would perform an ultrasound on my breast and give me news that could forever change my life and potentially end it.

I told Bob I was going to visit a friend who was having a bad day and cheer her up. Never had I been dishonest with Bob, and I felt terrible that day for doing so, but I simply couldn't tell him what was really happening. He would know the truth soon enough and understand why. I hoped that when I told him, it would be good news, something we could both exclaim, "Whew! That was close! So glad it was a false alarm." But in the meantime, the priority was him, his health and well-being, and I had to do whatever it took so that I didn't rock his boat.

Bob smiled. "You're just the best. You're always there for everyone. Everybody needs an Evelyn."

I laughed in response. "You're so cute. Do you know how much I love you?" I then threw my arms around him and probably held on a little longer than usual. "I'll be back soon. Until then, have a great day. Make sure to relax and have some fun. I'll see you in a few hours before you have to leave for the airport." Then I kissed him.

As much as I loved spending time with my husband, it was best he was leaving again so soon. His absence would give me the time I needed to contend with this situation without having to find another excuse to leave him again.

Hopefully, the next time he came home, this would be all behind me . . . behind us. Hopefully.

Hope was good, but that day, I felt that it had already said its goodbyes and left the building.

–29–

I Don't Belong Here

The trip to Cox Breast Clinic on Wednesday seemed so long. The more I drove toward downtown, the farther away I got from home.

Trying to be positive, I declared out loud, "What a beautiful day."

While pondering the blue skies, I then thought, *I should be home on this beautiful day, spending it with my husband before he has to go out of town again. I should not be heading downtown to spend this precious time inside some sterile building with a bunch of strangers.*

Like it or not, I didn't have an option, not if I needed answers. The closer I got to Cox Breast Clinic, the closer I got to the reality of what could potentially be happening inside my body.

Next thing I knew, I couldn't breathe again. My chest tightened as well as every muscle in my body.

People simply drove right by me. They were probably enjoying the beautiful day, not aware of the horror and pain that was going on in the driver's head next to them, and consequently, her body.

I found my destination and pulled into an empty spot. My stomach churned all the way through the parking lot and through the front doors.

Those inside smiled. A woman at the receptionist's desk greeted me in a friendly manner. "Welcome! How can I help you?"

I thought, *How about telling me I don't have breast cancer, and I'm not going to die.* Instead, I asked, "Could you please tell me where to go for my ultrasound?"

"Absolutely." She then gave me directions, pointing with her finger to add supporting visuals.

My mind kept screaming, *What am I doing here? I don't belong here!*

Thank goodness for her pointing because I couldn't process her words.

Once upstairs, another receptionist greeted me as well. "They'll be with you in just a moment."

She was right. I had just sat down when a nurse came to the waiting area. "Mrs. Kormondy, come right in." She led me to what looked like a store's fitting room. "You can use any of these empty changing rooms to get undressed from the waist up. Here's a gown you can put on. Make sure the opening's in the front. Then, you can sit in that waiting room, and we'll call you back shortly." She too used her finger to point to a second waiting room that I assumed was for those having mammograms and ultrasounds.

I took the gown from her and thought, *Wow, what a beautiful pink gown! And so soft.*

Then I stopped myself. Here I was, probably about to get some devastating news, and really, I get engrossed in the feel of a gown? Shrugging, I realized for once, that was a good thing; it got my mind off the present if only for a moment. Whether or not that was this clinic's intention, I appreciated how the gowns they provided could make a bad situation better for those facing breast cancer, giving them something soft and beautiful that can make them still feel pretty and feminine.

With the gown wrapped around me, I joined the other women in the designated waiting room. As soon as I entered, the air became stagnant, negating the room's warm colors and décor. Almost all the occupants wore the same robe as me. Some didn't appear concerned at all; they were probably there for routine mammograms. Others, on the other hand, appeared terrified as if they already knew their fate. Either way, no one spoke, no one smiled, no one even looked at each other. I couldn't remember when I had been in a more cold, terrifying atmosphere.

Those wearing regular clothes seemed to be a supporting friend or family member of some of the robe-clad occupants. I wished Bob were with me because I sure could have used his support. For now, however, that just wasn't going to happen.

All weekend, I hadn't told anyone, and here I sat all alone in this room of strangers, still keeping my condition, my thoughts, and my fear to myself. I simply didn't have the heart to dump another cancer diagnosis on my friends and family after everything they had done for us during Bob's battle with cancer, well, at least not until I had more information.

I pondered whether I should ask anyone to come back with me should I have to return. My heart started pounding hard again when I thought about *why* I would have to return, so I decided I would cross that bridge if I came to it.

The long wait to be called back for the ultrasound gave me too much time to think. But I didn't need to think; I needed hard-core answers.

Finally, I heard my named called. A young woman wearing hospital scrubs waited by the doorway with a file folder in her hand. After walking over to her, she introduced herself as the ultrasound technician and led me to a dimly lit room.

I lay on the table and opened my gown so that this technician could run the ultrasound wand over my breasts. The whole time, I stared at the ceiling, willing my mind to go somewhere happy. That place just evidently didn't exist at the time because I couldn't get my mind off the here and now.

Once the ultrasound ended, the tech gave me a towel to wipe off the gel she had applied to my chest for the test.

"You can go back to the waiting room," she instructed. "Someone will come to get you after the doctor reviews the results. Don't change out of your robe yet in case we need to do another ultrasound."

I nodded and did what I was told. Not knowing was the most excruciating part. As I joined the other robe-clad women, I realized that I was one of the terrified-looking ones in this room.

The same technician finally called my name again, and I left that cold room with relief but reminded myself where I was going—to get a definitive diagnosis or be told that everything was fine. My stomach started churning again.

The tech stood outside the same ultrasound room as before and then waved toward the door with her arm. "You can go back in there. The doctor will be here to see you in a few minutes."

How many times have I heard those words during the last couple of years? Then without any prompting, my mind went back in time again to Bob's experiences, and my heart raced all over again.

I can't go through that another time! I just can't, I pleaded in my head.

I climbed back onto the exam table and sat with my legs dangling on the side. Thankfully, the doctor interrupted my thoughts with her knock on the door. She entered with a warm smile, but still, she was hard to read as to what kind of news she bore.

She sat in a chair next to me. "Mrs. Kormondy,

your ultrasound shows a mass on your left breast. We need to look at it more extensively with a more intensive ultrasound as well as do a biopsy. We've scheduled an appointment for you to come back tomorrow so that we can go ahead and get those done."

I nodded. And no way was I coming back here alone!

I left, not knowing any more than what I did when I first arrived, only that my hard lump was actually a mass.

Did I or did I not have cancer? Can someone please tell me?

−30−

A More-Than-Likely Diagnosis

Seeing Bob off that afternoon was a blur. Somehow, I managed to keep my secret intact, but I didn't know how long I could keep up the charade. I needed him now so much but not as much as he needed the peace and calm to finish healing.

That night, I called my friend Kathy and told her what was happening. She was shocked at my news. "Evelyn, I'm so sorry to hear that you're going through this. How are you holding up? How is Bob holding up?"

"I'm okay," I sighed. "I just wish they would tell me one way or another if I have cancer, which is why I haven't told Bob anything yet. I don't want to say anything until I know for sure. I can't put him through a false alarm."

"Sure," Kathy agreed. "When will you know?"

"They scheduled an intensive ultrasound and biopsy for me for Thursday, which is tomorrow. Hopefully, they'll know something by then. Would you mind going with me? I would really appreciate the support."

She immediately responded, "Of course, I'll go with you, Evelyn. Just tell me what time." She was quiet a moment. "Maybe it's just a cyst or something."

"Maybe," I agreed, wanting her to be right, praying for her to be right.

We spoke a few minutes more, mainly about the logistics of the next day's appointment. Then I was left alone with my thoughts again, and oh how tormenting they were!

That night, I slept very little. Too many what-ifs invaded my thoughts. I just needed to know what I was facing, good or bad, so that I could move forward either way. But getting an answer dragged on and on.

The next morning, I picked Kathy up at her house, and we arrived at the hospital in plenty of time. After checking in, she went to the changing area with me. Then we sat together in the designated waiting room with all the other pink-robed ladies.

When my name was called, the tech told us that Kathy wasn't allowed to go back in the ultrasound area, so she stayed put.

"I'll be right here when you come back," she assured me with a smile.

Although this ultrasound was more intrusive, I rationalized that if this was what it took to get an answer, then so be it. Afterward, I walked back to the pink-robed room to wait with Kathy for the results. I had her to talk to, and that passed the time until I was called back again.

Unfortunately, Kathy still couldn't go with me because I was going back to the ultrasound area to see the doctor. My heart raced during the whole walk to the room and didn't let up while sitting on the exam table and waiting for the doctor.

The same doctor from the day before came in and pulled up a chair next to me. "Mrs. Kormondy, you definitely have a large mass, and it's more than likely cancer. I'm sorry." She paused and studied my response, her eyes showing compassion.

It felt as if a bucket of cold water just got dumped on me. Although I tried to prepare myself for these words, I don't think anyone could be completely ready to hear that they had cancer, even if it was more than likely.

"More than likely? So you're not sure," I pointed out.

The doctor shifted in her chair. "Mrs. Kormondy, between what we're seeing in the ultrasound and your family history, we're pretty sure it's breast cancer. I want to go ahead and do a biopsy now. It's quick. We're also going to need bloodwork. We're sending you to an oncologist, a surgeon, and also a radiation oncologist. Regardless of what it turns out to be, we're confident enough that something's going on, and you need to see a surgeon."

Well, at least I had my answer . . . sort of. Still, "more than likely cancer" and "pretty sure it's cancer" didn't sound like "for-sure cancer."

"So let's get started with a biopsy," she said.

A nurse appeared out of nowhere with a tray containing medical stuff.

The doctor took something off it and started rubbing it on my breast. "First, I'm applying something here to numb your skin," she explained as she felt the lump. "Then I'll need to make a small incision over the area where I'll be inserting a needle to remove a sample of the tissue."

I nodded. "I understand. I watched as my husband went through biopsies."

As promised, the procedure was quick. Perhaps one reason was because I wasn't paying attention to what she was doing to my breast but was focused on my "more than likely" diagnosis.

She started removing her gloves. "This is an order for bloodwork." She handed me a piece of paper. "Before you leave, please go downstairs to the lab and get it done. Tomorrow, you'll need to come back. We'll assign a guide to you to walk you through everything . . . the plan, the next steps, and she'll take you to meet each of the doctors. They can tell you themselves what to expect."

I nodded and left to get dressed. Progress had been made, but it wasn't good progress. At least I learned it was "more than likely cancer." The unknown was starting to become clearer, and I didn't like it; in fact, I was terrified of it. I had looked that monster in the eye three times before (once in my own body and twice in Bob's), but the last time almost took me down.

Fear and depression merged as I contemplated my future. After getting my blood drawn, I walked to the main waiting room to meet Kathy.

Her raised eyebrows and smile quickly vanished as soon as she saw me. She didn't say one word. We walked through the parking lot in silence. There were no words that would come out of my mouth as I tried to process the doctor's report.

Once we were both in the quiet of my car, I placed my hands on the steering wheel and stared straight ahead. "Kathy, according to the doctor, the mass I have in my breast is more than likely cancer." I couldn't say that "c" word without breaking down and crying.

Kathy reached over and pulled me to her as we cried together. "If it is cancer, Evelyn, you'll beat it!" she encouraged me with resolve.

"Yes," I responded, not quite sure I sounded as confident as her, so I gave it another try, this time with more force. "Yes, I *will* beat this cancer."

– 3 1 –

Why? Why? Why?

Here I was again, repeating perpetual medical appointments. But this time, I went to them alone. Bob still didn't know, and although the doctor felt that it was "more than likely cancer," I still couldn't tell him.

I had to first wrap it all around my own head and pull myself together so that when I told him, I wouldn't fall apart. I knew I would probably crumble anyway, and Bob would be my rock as he has always been. He would hold me and tell me everything was going to be okay.

However, he had just started to breathe again, to get his life back on track. I couldn't go and push him off it when I didn't know for sure. To me, there was a chance, although a small one, that it wasn't cancer.

We both knew all too well that when cancer struck, everyone close by was hit by it as well. It was even more devastating within a couple. When cancer happened to one of us, it happened to us both. When Bob had cancer, my world revolved around it even though I didn't directly have it. Now, Bob's world would be turned upside down again and revolve around my cancer. Until then, I would pray and gather my strength from God.

So on Friday morning, God and I returned to the breast center where they assigned a guide to take me through what I needed to do and what to expect.

The guide took me to see the oncologist. I didn't like him. He wanted to start giving me chemo immediately without knowing more about what we were dealing with, and he couldn't answer my questions. I had no confidence in him and didn't want to use his services.

Then she took me to see a surgeon. Although he was better than the oncologist, I wasn't comfortable with him either. Maybe it was simply my fear, but I didn't want to use his services either.

Next on our tour was the plastic surgeon, Dr. Andrew Paine, and I liked him. He came across as informative and caring, a great choice for my complete double mastectomy. But the fact that I only liked one out of three doctors made me rethink Cox Breast Clinic.

All weekend, I still didn't say anything to Bob; he was working. Instead, I contemplated the doctors I met, and the whole thing felt wrong. They were ready to put me through a whole lot of stuff, and they didn't yet know any of the details.

Maybe I shouldn't stay at Cox. Perhaps Mercy had an oncologist and surgeon with whom I could feel comfortable. They had been so kind to Bob, and they had earned my trust and confidence.

Monday morning, I called Dr. Simpson since he was our friend, and we trusted him. Maybe he could be my doctor. If not, then at least he had privileges at Mercy, so he would know their doctors and which were good and which weren't.

His staff told me that they didn't treat breast cancer. I wasn't surprised, but it was worth a shot. Fortunately, Mercy had other doctors who could. They referred me to a surgeon, an oncologist, and a radiation oncologist.

I made the decision to go ahead and make an appointment with their surgeon Dr. Ginger Stevens. I had nothing to lose but everything to gain—my life—if it was the right fit. So I took her first available appointment, which happened to be the next Monday, one week from that day. Bob would be out of town again. I wanted him there, but it was what it was, and I couldn't wait any longer to start treatment.

Later that day, the lady who scheduled my appointment called to inform me that before Dr. Stevens could see me, she wanted me to get more blood work. She put in an order to a lab close to me.

I went to the lab first thing in the morning, and I was impressed when I saw everything she had marked off on the order, more than what Cox had asked for. She seemed very thorough, as if she was checking for everything possible and digging deep so that she could find out what was really going on with me. So far, so good.

Bob's plane would be landing soon, so I put on some makeup to greet him. Looking at my reflection in the mirror, it still didn't cover up the stress.

While waiting for Bob to come home from the airport, all I could focus on was my telling him about my cancer. My treatments would be starting too soon, and I could no longer put off telling him. He needed to get involved, meet my doctors, and give me his advice, but I still didn't know what to say. How would he react? Where would he get the strength to handle this horrible and shocking news?

He was working so hard on getting back what cancer had taken from him, and some things he had lost forever. Plus, he was trying to take care of his family and himself. Now, I had to tell him this news.

Dear God, how do I do this? He is such a good man. Why?

Why? Why? Why? A question that kept reverberating in my brain. Regardless, I had to move forward, and I needed him with me. He had a right to know now and before he left again to go back to work.

Seeing his face as he walked into our family room still made my heart skip a beat. Thankfully, he was too far away to hear the small gasp that escaped from me as I contemplated his reaction when I told him. No way was I going to hit him with it at this time. The right moment would come; I would know it. Then and only then would I say something to him.

What was important was that we enjoyed our time together as always. I allowed myself to live in the moment as I tried to stay focused on him instead of my plight.

That night as we got ready for bed, I felt it was the right time, so I took advantage of a pause in our conversation.

"Bob, I have something to tell you," I began.

"What, honey?" he asked in a happy voice as if I was about to tell him some exciting news.

Poor guy. He had no idea what he was about to be hit with, so I tried to give him a heads-up so that he could first brace himself, although it probably wouldn't be enough.

My throat started constricting, and I wasn't sure if I could speak. Bob waited patiently.

Finally, I managed to say, "It's not good, honey, but I know God will help us."

His smile and that twinkle in his eyes that I loved so much disappeared. His eyebrows furrowed in concern. "What is it, Evie?"

Tears formed in my eyes. "Something's wrong with me."

He studied me for a moment. "What are you talking about?"

"The Saturday when you were at the U.S. Open, I felt a lump in my breast." I couldn't help it; I started to cry.

Tears now starting pooling in his eyes. "Well, maybe it's nothing, darling. Let's pray."

We did, and then I finished telling him the news.

"I've already had some tests, Bob, so it is something. The doctors seem confident it's breast cancer."

His eyes popped open wide in shock, and he didn't speak for a few moments. Finally, he proclaimed, "Well, then we'll get a second opinion."

I nodded in agreement, and we both cried together.

Then he asked the same questions as me when I first learned about it—"Why is this happening? I don't understand. I just got well. There's no way this could be happening to our family again! Our life is lining up, and now, the love of my life is sick. I don't understand what's happening. Please, God, help us!"

"He will help us," I affirmed. "I've been praying for guidance and where I should be treated. I don't feel comfortable with Cox Breast Clinic. I don't feel they did enough testing."

Bob nodded. "Then you shouldn't go there. You shouldn't be treated by any doctor you're not comfortable with. What are you going to do now?"

"Well, Mercy was so good to you, so I called Dr. Simpson's office today. They recommended another surgeon at Mercy named Dr. Stevens. She would be doing my mastectomy. I have an appointment with her on Monday. Bob, I want you there with me; I need you there with me. We can talk to her together and see if she's a fit. We can find out together what needs to be done so that we can understand it, and I can get started with the treatments."

He nodded and hugged me. "Absolutely, Evie! Of course, I'll go with you. I want to know what's going on, exactly what they're going to do to you, and what we can expect. I'll be there with you just like you were there with me to support me. I'll call work in the morning and cancel my next trip."

I was so relieved and thankful because I needed to rely on his strength. I was the one who helped sick family members, but when it came to my being sick, I couldn't handle it. Only with God and Bob would I be able to take this day by day.

−32−

Definitely Not a Quick Fix

Over the next couple of days, Bob and I prayed a lot and went to the beach, which was both our sanctuary and our playground. We tried to let loose and lighten up the seriousness of my situation and relieve some of the pent-up stress. Then we walked a bit along the water's edge and talked about what we thought needed to be done to get ahead of the doctors.

He held me as the waves lapped against our ankles. How I had craved that strength, that protectiveness. I held onto him, not wanting to let go.

We loosened our grips, and Bob stepped back and looked deeply into my eyes. "Evie, you are so strong. You can do this."

His endorsement and belief in me were encouraging. At this point, every bit helped.

Afterwards, Bob drove me to Cox Breast Clinic to pick up my records. Having him with me this time as we approached the building gave me confidence and peace. He was with me and by my side now. Together, we were a formidable force.

We then drove to Dr. Stevens's office to give her my records so that she could be familiar with my case before we met. Bob could have waited in the car while I rushed in to drop them off, but he wanted to walk inside with me. I guess for him, that was one step closer to engaging himself in my treatment.

Then much too soon yet not soon enough, Bob drove me to my appointment with Dr. Stevens. She was tall with blond hair, light blue eyes, and a warm demeanor. I liked her immediately.

After talking with us for a few minutes, I felt exceptionally confident in her abilities. Then she said, "Mrs. Kormondy, I've gone through all your records, and I'm fairly certain you have stage 3 triple-negative breast cancer."

That word "negative" can really throw a person into thinking it's a good thing. We had been so used to hearing that word from Bob's doctors where it meant that you didn't have the condition. As a result, our initial reaction was excitement.

"It's negative! That's great!" Bob responded and smiled at me. "So she doesn't have breast cancer after all!"

The doctor didn't share our enthusiasm. "No, Mr. Kormondy. That is not good. That's actually a diagnosis of an extremely aggressive form of breast cancer."

Her last words devastated us and stopped us in our tracks.

Aggressive cancer? That's exactly what they said about Bob's cancer, and he had to go through a lot to be more aggressive to survive it. They said if he didn't go through their prescribed treatment plans, he had only four months to live.

Taking in a deep breath and then letting it out, I asked, "What needs to be done next, Dr. Stevens? Surgery?" Since Bob started off his cancer treatment with surgery, I just figured that's how mine would start.

"Stage 3 triple-negative is too aggressive, and the mass is too large for surgery right now," she responded. "In the meantime, I've ordered a PET scan for you and made an appointment for you on Wednesday with the oncologist. Her name is Dr. Brandi Carson. She'll talk to you about the chemotherapy treatments and schedule."

My brain wasn't keeping up with the doctor's rapid fire of bad news. It hadn't finished processing her first round before she fired another one at us. At this point, I simply couldn't speak. Frankly, it was all l could do to not get up and run to the restroom and throw up.

Dr. Stevens explained, "Again, it's a large mass, Mrs. Kormondy, so we need to first shrink the tumor with chemotherapy before we can go in and operate and try to get it all. Even though the cancer's on the left side, it's best to go ahead and have a radical double mastectomy due to your family history and the diagnosis of stage 3 triple-negative breast cancer."

I nodded in agreement. I had already resigned myself to the fact that I would need to have both of my breasts completely removed, go through chemotherapy, radiation, and then reconstruction surgery. It all sounded ominous and definitely not a quick fix, more serious and terrifying than I had anticipated.

Dear Lord, how long is this going to take? Am I going to survive and be there for Bob, the love of my life?

During our drive home, neither of us spoke. We were in shock. We had thought that Mercy, chemo, and radiation were all behind us. How could this be happening again? How could we go through this again?

I could only imagine what was going through Bob's head, wondering how he would be able to go through this with me while he tries to work. He had been trying to pay off his medical bills, and now, he would need to support the massive cost of my medical care.

I knew my husband and that it wasn't about the money; it was about his wife, about both of us being alive. Still, we were heading into more debt, and that ultimately fell onto Bob.

When we got home, we went for a walk. We held hands and discussed everything he had experienced and how he had come out of it alive.

He encouraged me again. "Evie, you can do this. You can get to the other side too. In the meantime, just like you told me when I was going through cancer, we'll take it day by day and leave tomorrow on the calendar where it belongs. We'll take every moment we can and know that's the only way to get to the other side. It's day by day."

His words empowered me as they resounded in my mind. They reminded of the song "Day by Day" from the musical film *Godspell* back in the '70s. The song's words were classic, and they resonated with me and the journey upon which I was about to embark.

From then on, I would make "Day by Day" my anthem.

−33−

Reporting for Duty

I couldn't believe I was about to enter another battle a mere fifteen months after my husband had finished his. I hadn't even recuperated from fighting his neck and throat cancer, and now, here I was again, fighting my own cancer. The only thing I brought with me to the battlefield was experience. And with that experience came the fear from knowing too much about the intensity that was sure to follow.

It tore Bob up for him to have to return to work a couple of days after Dr. Stevens gave us the diagnosis of stage 3 triple-negative breast cancer. He was such a source of emotional strength when home, but he had missed so much work through his own ordeal. Not only were we without his income (as well as mine), but we still were addressing the medical debt that had been incurred from his treatments. Frankly, we both felt the pressure of needing the money.

I tried to take away his guilt. "Bob, sweetheart, it's just my first treatment," I encouraged. "And I'm not going through radiation at the same time like you did. It's just chemo, so I'll be okay. I'll get a friend to go with me, and you'll be home in a couple of days anyway. Go! I'll be fine."

Actually, I didn't feel so fine; just the contrary—I was frightened! Everyone kept telling me, "You have to do this, Evelyn. You have to . . . you have to!"

I obviously had no choice in the matter and thus, no control. Honestly, it made me feel trapped and claustrophobic. At times, it made breathing difficult. So, I would have to stop and then center and remind myself that in the whole big scheme of things, it was for a short time.

You can do this, Evelyn!

I started this journey thinking my treatment plan would be similar to Bob's—double mastectomy surgery to remove the cancer followed by chemo and radiation concurrently. I didn't like having something lethal growing inside me. As far as I was concerned, I just wanted the cancer out of me, and the sooner the better.

According to Dr. Stevens, it didn't work that way.

Bob and I had different cancers, and they had to be addressed accordingly. Because of the type of cancer I had and its large tumor size, there was a very high percentage of it returning.

Enter Dr. Carson, my oncologist, an intelligent and kind woman. Just like with Dr. Stevens, I felt comfortable with her and her knowledge and competency, and as time went on, she would prove herself to be a hands-on oncologist—always returning phone calls, answering questions in simplistic terms, and there for me overall. I felt her sincere care.

Whereas Dr. Stevens was the head doctor and sent orders to the other doctors for what needed to be done, Dr. Carson responded to those orders and stepped in to treat me using her specialty. She was responsible for ensuring I had the appropriate medications, including the chemo drugs.

During our first appointment, she explained my treatment plan, echoing Dr. Stevens: the chemotherapy will shrink the tumor so that it could be removed during surgery later on.

"I've ordered six chemotherapy treatments for you, Evelyn," she stated.

"How often do I have them?" I asked. Bob had one every few days, so I should be finished with them rather quickly. That would be great! Just get it done!

She looked at her paperwork. "You will have one treatment every three weeks. The first one starts one week from today, on July 10."

The nurse handed me a printout that contained a list of dates and times for when I was to have my chemotherapy. Of course, my eyes travelled to the last one—October 30. I would have preferred to finish them much sooner, but I guess spreading them out over fifteen weeks wasn't too bad.

I left the office that day with my marching orders in hand. In one week, the process of first and foremost shrinking the tumor as much as possible would begin. As both doctors emphasized, the more they shrunk the tumor, the more chance they would have to get all of the cancer and the less chance it would have to spread more, and the less chance I would need to have more treatments and even another surgery. Shrinking the tumor first via chemo would also make it easier to remove my breasts and lymph nodes during the surgery.

Of course, the battle would still be on because even after all that, I could still have cancer floating around inside me. I could get metastatic breast cancer where it could metastasize or spread to other parts of my body, like my bones, lungs and other organs, or even my brain, and that is not curable. So after all this, I would have to go through radiation because the doctors wanted to eradicate it the best they could and as much as possible.

Notwithstanding, the bottom line was that there was always a chance of the cancer coming back, ergo my doctors' very aggressive treatment plan. Bite the bullet now and be rewarded with life. I didn't like it, but all three types of treatments and procedures were the best plan of action with cancers that rapidly reproduce and spread. I had gone through all of them with Bob, and now, I would go through all of them myself.

The waiting was difficult. I figured I had a good idea of what to expect, such as the hair loss for which chemo and radiation had earned a well-deserved reputation. So on one hand, I dreaded the fight. But on the other hand, I wanted to get it over with and behind me so that I could move on with my life.

Regardless, I could almost sense the cancer within my body challenging me to a duel. Preparation was essential in minimizing the damage. So I sharpened my tools by getting on my knees and praying, reading the Bible, and praising God through music. I was determined to be victorious!

About two weeks before I started chemotherapy, I had an appointment with Dr. Stevens. She said, "We've got you scheduled for June 26 at the outpatient surgical center to implant a medical port device."

"A medical what?" I asked.

Dr. Stevens smiled. "A medical port. It's a small medical device we'll insert under your skin on the upper right side of your chest. It'll make it easier when you have your chemo treatments and other IVs, even getting blood drawn. That way, we don't have to stick you each time and blow out your veins. During treatments, we'll just need to insert the IV line into the port, and the chemo will be able to run directly into your body."

"Under the skin? Will it hurt? I asked.

"Nah," she responded. "When you come to the surgical center, we'll put you in a twilight sleep, and then when you wake up, it'll be all over. You may feel a little discomfort a day or two afterwards, but most people are fine."

Surgical center?

"But neither of my sisters who had breast cancer had a port. My husband Bob didn't have a port either, and he had seven chemo treatments. I only have six, and they're scheduled much farther apart," I argued.

Dr. Stevens shrugged. "Evelyn, I wasn't involved in your sisters' and your husband's treatments, but their veins could have been much stronger."

I nodded, trying to process her words. Sounded logical. I didn't recall anything about my sisters' veins, but I did know that Bob had tremendously strong veins. Thinking back to that time, though, I remembered that all his treatments weren't easy on him and his veins.

I decided I would rather do it this way with the port. Again, bite the bullet now so I wouldn't have to be stuck with more needles than necessary.

Dr. Stevens had her staff schedule me for the procedure. In my mind, having a port inserted wasn't "committing" myself to this whole battle thing; it was just preparing in case I decided to do it.

Despite all of the reports and test results, I was still having a difficult time wrapping my head around my having cancer and that I would have to fight the fight of my life. It's hard to imagine that you're *terminally ill* when you feel fine, even great!

So on the set date and time, my dad drove me to the surgical center for the port. After checking and recording my vitals, I was taken to a small surgical room and given an IV. Within moments, I started drifting off. Frankly, I don't remember when I fell asleep; I just remember opening my eyes and looking around the curtained area and figuring out where I was.

Oh yeah, I just had my port implanted, I thought.

I felt the port under my skin, but it didn't hurt one bit. I shrugged, feeling pretty proud of myself for taking this so well. After all, they had just installed a piece of gear to better equip me for battle.

When July 10 arrived at the infusion center, I "reported for duty" as a good soldier does. I had asked my friend Sophie if she could drive me. Without hesitation, she agreed.

We arrived at Mercy in plenty of time for my first chemotherapy appointment. When my name was called to go back for the treatment, I looked over at Sophie. She gave me a quick nod and smiled encouragingly at me.

"Evelyn," she said, "I'll be right here praying for you."

I felt her strength, and it propelled me to take a first step.

You can do this, Evelyn! I encouraged myself.

The nurse smiled warmly and led me into a large, quiet room full of women sitting in recliners and connected to IV poles via clear plastic tubing. Almost everyone in those chairs wore turbans or wigs to cover their bald heads caused by the very thing that was flooding through their veins at the time.

The nurse then pointed to a recliner. "You can sit here, Mrs. Kormondy. Make yourself comfortable."

I stared at that recliner for a few moments before taking her up on her offer. To me, that chair represented the battlefield, and I wasn't quite ready to step onto it. Then I realized I may never be ready.

Taking a deep breath, I slowly sat down. As a result, I knew in that moment, I had fully engaged in the battle.

−34−

The Red Devil

The recliner turned out to be very comfortable, but it did nothing to calm my fear.

Within moments, an older woman with graying hair wrapped in a bun on top of her head came over to me. The nurse introduced her to me as Carmen and added, "You're in good hands with her, Mrs. Kormondy."

I nodded, praying she was right. The nurse left, and Carmen began setting me up with my treatment. She explained everything as she did it, hanging up several medication bags on the IV pole. Her warm, caring, and gentle demeanor made me like and trust her immediately.

"What are all these medications?" I asked. "There are so many of them."

She smiled in understanding and told me the name of each as she pointed to them. One bag contained a red liquid. "This one's called the 'red devil,'" she said.

A shudder went through my body. No way were they putting something into me called red devil.

"I don't like that name," I responded. "Please call it 'God's angel of healing.' Please never refer to it as the 'red devil' when I'm getting it."

Carmen nodded and smiled warmly. "I can do that, Mrs. Kormondy," she assured me optimistically and then added, "I'm only giving you 90 percent of your treatments."

Interesting, I thought.

"Why 90 percent?" I asked.

"Well, we don't want to overwhelm you. Let's get you started so that you can be eased into it," she answered patiently and kindly while rubbing an alcohol pad to disinfect the port area.

Eased into it? I didn't like the sound of that.

After successfully sanitizing the port, Carmen inserted the needle from the IV tubing into my port. She said, "Okay, Mrs. Kormondy, everything's good to go. Just sit back and relax."

Yep, here we go, I thought. *Here I am, sitting in this nice comfortable chair, baring my port. Time to put the poison into my body, and I'm allowing it to happen. There's no turning back now.*

It was a surreal moment of watching the poison making its way through the clear IV's tubing until it finally reached its destination—my port, which gave it complete and total access into my body.

It was a strong reality check, and I forced myself not to cry out loud as I contemplated what was truly happening. Many of the others seemed to be comfortable while receiving their chemo, and I didn't want to scare or disturb them. So I settled upon allowing the tears to flow freely down my cheeks.

Remember, Evelyn, this poison is killing the cancer, not you, I reminded myself.

And then, the tubing remained full of that poisoned liquid, and I knew it would continue until they decided to stop it. I had no more control at this point.

To get through the emotional impact, I meditated on Bob's words, which were the same words I had told him during his cancer treatments: "You are stronger than cancer. Let me repeat . . . you are stronger than cancer!"

"How long does this take?" I asked, tilting my head toward the IV bags.

"About three hours." Carmen looked on my lap where I had laid a paperback book. "Oh good. I see you've brought something to read. Let me know if you need something, Mrs. Kormondy." Then she walked away.

I opened my book, but my eyes were so full of tears that I couldn't read it. All I could think about were those medications going into my body. Were they going to heal me or hurt me? Would they make me sick? I didn't know the answers to any of these questions, and that scared me more.

Then every thirty to forty-five minutes or so, Carmen would come back and change the IV bags with new ones.

By the third round, I asked, "How much of the red God's angel of healing do I have to take?

She kept her focus on the unhooking and rehooking of the IV tubing. "Today, you're getting five bags."

My eyes popped wide open in shock. *Five bags?*

When it was over, Sophie drove me home. Fortunately, I wouldn't have to return for three weeks. One down, five to go . . .

And for right now, chemotherapy was out of sight, out of mind, in the rearview mirror as I would think after Bob's treatments. Those now seemed a lifetime ago while simultaneously feeling like they were still fresh.

Sophie glanced over at me from the driver's seat. "How do you feel, Evelyn? You okay?"

I nodded. "I feel okay now, but I don't know how I'll feel later, what to expect. I'm pretty nervous about that."

She reached over and gently patted my hand. "Why don't I just spend the night, just in case?"

I let out a sigh of relief. "That would be great. Thank you!"

As soon as I entered my house, I rushed to my bedroom to change into some comfortable clothes. Then I joined Sophie in the family room to watch TV and get my mind off everything. Hopefully, we would simply have a girl's night of watching funny movies and eating popcorn.

For the next hour, I lay on the couch, enjoying Sophie's company. Then, nausea overwhelmed me so much that my stomach hurt. Sophie helped me to the bathroom where I proceeded to get very sick. My head hurt as well as my whole body.

I didn't expect such a horrific physical response and so quickly. Maybe I had been thinking about radiation and how it had a cumulative effect, that a person didn't start feeling its consequences until after it had saturated their body from numerous treatments. Obviously, I had severely miscalculated what my chemotherapy treatments could do . . . and when.

Sophie bent down to help me up and to my bedroom.

I mumbled, "I can't. I can't. I don't have the energy."

I then lay on the bathroom floor, and she covered me up with a towel. I cried, I was so sick and truly felt like I was dying.

Thank God Sophie was there. Just having her presence brought me comfort in the midst of one of the worst nights I had ever experienced thus far. My body had rebelled horribly at what it just got injected with.

But I had five more. If my body reacted this badly to the first treatment, I couldn't help but wonder what it would do after the next ones.

−35−

The Chemo Fog

Why can't my brain wake up? Even walking to the bathroom didn't affect my light-headedness. Usually, a good cup of coffee would wake it up, but my queasy stomach from the night before dismissed the idea.

My cell phone rang, and I looked at the screen to see who it was. I didn't recognize the number, but at this point, my brain was too foggy. It could be important, so I answered it anyway.

"Hello?"

"Mrs. Kormondy?" a voiced asked on the other end. "This is the infusion center. I'm calling to see how you're doing."

How was I doing? Boy, that was a loaded question! How much time do you have? Somehow my brain was able to conjure up that much.

Instead, I spoke, "I'm okay, I guess. Last night was rough, actually, horrible, but I think I'm better now." I then proceeded to tell her some of the details of what I had experienced.

The caller sounded sympathetic to my plight. "That's not uncommon," she commented. "I'm sorry you went through that." She then encouraged me to call the infusion center or my doctor if my symptoms got worse.

I assured her I would as we told each other bye. I then scanned my phone to check my texts, but those that had come in, their words didn't make sense.

Sophie came into my bedroom. "Evelyn, how are you feeling? Do you think you could eat a little something?"

My stomach wasn't willing to accept food either. I shook my head with a weak smile. "Thanks, Sophie, but I don't think eating anything right now would be a good idea. I'm still very nauseous. Also, thank you for being here with me last night. I'm feeling much better . . . a little weak, but we have to go back to the infusion center for them to give me that IV for dehydration and shot for nausea. I don't feel like it, but I must be dehydrated after all that happened last night, and I sure could use something for the nausea. So, I need to make myself get up and get ready. In the meantime, I'm just trying to shake out the cobwebs in my brain."

"Well," she responded, "You were very sick last night. Who wouldn't have cobwebs after all that?" She paused and studied me for a moment. "You'll feel so much better after the shot and IV. Do you need me to help you get dressed? I can then drive you there whenever you're ready."

"I'm going to try to get dressed by myself. Give me a few minutes to change, and then we can work on walking to the car." I chuckled from the little bit of humor I found in envisioning that scenario.

Sophie left the room so I could get dressed. I made it out of bed and to my closet, but as I stared at my hanging clothes, it didn't take long to realize that what I was experiencing was more than cobwebs; it was a fog. I couldn't think without confusion; nothing made sense. I couldn't concentrate nor could I clearly remember much. It was as if I was watching the world from the outside.

Then it dawned on me—Bob had expressed the same challenges when he went through chemotherapy. People would laugh it off and call it "chemo brain" or "chemo fog." Well, I found out that when going through it, it wasn't so funny and nothing to joke about. It was frustrating and scary because I couldn't force my brain to operate like it previously had.

Recognizing it as temporary made me feel better while at the same time, it daunted me to know it was one more thing to deal with for the next several months.

You'll get through this, Evelyn. You will, I encouraged myself. *You* need *to get through this. You're strong.* I then prayed for God to help me.

I picked out something to wear, but I wasn't quite sure it made sense, nor did I care. I ran a brush through my hair and stared in the mirror at my pale face and dark circles under my bloodshot eyes.

Sophie was waiting for me in the kitchen. She held my elbow as we walked to her car. Her touch was light, so her hand was really there to provide more of an emotional support than physical.

I was so glad I went. Once I took the anti-nausea shot and had the IV, I felt so much better. Sophie drove me home afterward and helped me get inside my house and into my bed.

I felt guilty taking up so much of her time, but I surely did appreciate it. "Sophie," I said, "I know you need to get home. I'll be okay by myself now. I'm going to rest, and then Bob will be home tomorrow."

She gave a reluctant nod as she studied me with skepticism. "Okay, but call me if you need anything."

I nodded and then thanked her again. The door closed in the background, and I was alone. Soon afterward, sleep mercifully came upon me where I was grateful I didn't have to think.

The next morning, I woke up encouraged. Bob was coming home! He would again be taking a cab from the airport, and I couldn't wait to see him! With him here, I would be better. He would take care of me. Most importantly, he would strengthen me.

He would also help me think. But until then, I couldn't even decide what to wear. Should I take a shower now or wait? Then I couldn't figure out what I should do first—take a shower or choose what to wear, or should I straighten the bed? None of it made sense.

I had always taken pride in my decision-making and organizational skills, but now, I would start one task, and before completing it, I would go on to another. Now both skills had become downright impaired at best but more like paralyzed.

Thankfully, I managed to take a shower, get dressed, and straighten the bed a few minutes before Bob walked through the front door.

Sitting in our family room, my eyes stayed fixed on the entryway from our living room. Then I saw him, and boy, what a sight he was!

He rushed over to me on the love seat and greeted me with a huge smile. "How you feelin', Evie?"

I returned his smile. "Better now that you're here!" I didn't want to dump my complaints on him as soon as he came home.

He hugged me again and kissed the top of my head. Bob was sensitive to the aftermath of chemo. He knew I would be wiped out, so he did most of the talking for the rest of the day. He shared stories and events about his trip and the tournament he worked, and I was glad for the opportunity to stay quiet.

I couldn't think of much to say anyway. Even if I did, it probably wouldn't have made much sense.

−36−

The Loss of Losing My Hair

Bob waited on me, bringing me whatever I needed, and he encouraged me to rest so I that could regain my strength.

It worked. Slowly but surely, I was walking around at a normal pace. It was hard to reconcile the way I felt now with how I had felt a few nights earlier.

Even though it seemed like I was getting back to the old Evie, I still needed Bob. Unfortunately, he was scheduled to leave again in another two days, and this time for Lake Tahoe for the annual American Century Celebrity Golf Championship Tournament. I dreaded his leaving. Plus, this tournament happened to be one of my favorites.

So I came up with an idea and approached him with it that evening. "Bob, we've only got a couple of days left together before you have to leave again. I miss you. I'm doing so much better, and I'll be doing even better by the time you leave. So I want to go with you to Lake Tahoe. It'll be a much-needed distraction for me. It'll be good break. I'll get on the plane, and then when we get there, I'll just look at the lake. You know how much I love to do that. It'll also give me a chance to see my friends who work with you." I stopped and grinned sheepishly. "Okay, they're really your friends," I admitted, "but they're really nice to me."

Bob didn't come back with his usual excitement when I told him I wanted to go on a trip with him. Instead, he studied me for a moment. "Evie, are you sure? You know I love having you with me, but are you sure you're up to it?"

I smiled because at that moment, I was up to it! No nausea. "I feel wonderful! I feel absolutely normal. I must have gotten it all out of my system that first night. Have you noticed that I'm sleeping through the night and haven't gotten sick one time since you've been home?"

He continued pondering me as I continued smiling at him. "Okay then," he said, "let's go to Tahoe!"

That night, I started packing my bags. I was so excited, not only to go to Lake Tahoe and spend that time with Bob, but this trip also represented my ability to continue on with my life despite the cancer. Through it, I was telling cancer that it wouldn't, couldn't get me down; it had no power over me. I was going to show it who was boss. After all, I popped back rather quickly from that ghastly night after my first treatment. I was back to the same ole Evie.

But the next morning, I woke up to find hair all over my pillow. Realizing that was my hair and that the chemo was already causing it to fall out, I rushed to the bathroom in shock to see how much I had left, if any.

Horrified, I stared at myself in the mirror. *Oh no! My beautiful red hair!* It had been just like my mom's hair, and it was one thing I was hoping to keep.

I didn't want to disturb Bob, so I got into the shower, turned the water on full blast, and bawled.

My hair! I loved my hair!

Bob walked into the bathroom. "You okay in there?"

Forcing my cries to stop, I answered, "Yes. I'm fine. I guess you saw the hair on my pillow."

"I did. I'm so sorry, Evie. There's nothing I can do to stop this effect, but I truly wish I could. It happens sooner or later, whether it's chemo or radiation, but remember, it's temporary. You'll have your gorgeous red hair back before you know it."

"Well, it happened sooner," I replied between sniffles. "I'll be out in a few minutes."

After drying off, I put the brush to my head and paused, pretty sure more would fall out with the process. Taking a deep breath, I whispered, "Here goes" and gently brushed my hair from the scalp to the ends.

I got dressed and went to the kitchen to make a cup of coffee. Bob was sitting on the couch watching the news. When he heard me come in, he turned and gave me a reassuring smile. He picked up the remote from the coffee table and clicked off the TV.

He walked over to me, and I placed my hands over my head. He took both my wrists and pulled my hands away. "You look beautiful," he said and gave me a tight hug.

"Since I'm losing hair," I started, trying not to break down again, "I guess I'm going to need to pack some scarves to cover the bald spots while we're in Tahoe. I don't want anyone to see them."

Losing my hair was going to happen, like it or not. When Bob went through chemotherapy, the doctors told him that while the chemo killed the cancer, it would also kill other things too, like hair follicles. Fortunately, Bob lost very little hair. His hair loss came from the radiation. It looked as if someone had taken a buzz razor and shaved the back of his head from one end to the other. Eventually, it did grow back to a full head of hair.

At least I would have Bob with me to assure me. So I went into our closet to go through my scarf collection and choose ones that matched my outfits.

The next morning, I woke up to more hair loss. In my mind, I tried to adjust to it, telling myself that it was part of the process, but admittedly, I wasn't doing a good job.

In the midst of my grieving, my neighbor Nita called. She could hear I was upset over the phone, so I broke down and told her about my hair loss.

"Oh, Evelyn. I'm so sorry," she lamented with me.

Not long after we hung up, she called back, her voice enthusiastic. "Evelyn," she started, "I'm buying you a wig today before you leave tomorrow on your trip!"

I couldn't let her do that. "No, that's okay, Nita. I appreciate your offering, though."

"Please let me do this," she insisted. "Please. It'll be

fun. That way, you can go to Tahoe and feel gorgeous. I want to be part of making that happen!"

"Well, if you're sure," I consented.

Thank God, Nita was of the mindset that even warriors on the battlefield still needed to feel pretty.

She picked me up in her car, even though she just lived next door. It would have been an easy stroll, but she drove her car one house over and parked it in my driveway to cause me as little effort as possible.

Admittedly, I was excited. Regardless of the fact that I was going shopping for a wig, I was still embarrassed about the bald areas. So I wore a scarf to cover them.

Nita drove me to a wonderful wig shop that she had found online that worked with cancer patients. Once there, I removed my scarf so that the shopkeeper could see my real hair, or what was left of it.

"I think I have the perfect wig for you!" she exclaimed with a big grin and scurried off.

She came back with a beautiful red wig that was long. It reminded me of my hair. When I put it on, I felt so pretty.

Nita observed my reaction. "We'll take it," she announced to the shopkeeper. Then she purchased it for me. I will never forget her act of kindness.

Now I had something that didn't scream to the world that I had cancer. I had hair again! Granted, it wasn't my hair, but it was my wig that looked like my hair.

Cancer may have won this battle, but it would not win this war! That victory belonged to God. My role was to do my part and leave the rest up to Him.

−37−

Lake Tahoe,
Here We Come Again

It was about a six-hour flight. I slept through most of it, but I was still glad when we landed.

We stepped off the plane in the Sacramento International Airport, and I still felt fine. So far so good. See, this cancer thing wasn't going to stop me!

Full of confidence, I climbed into our rented car to start our fifty-three-mile, two-hour drive on a windy road to our hotel in Stateline, Nevada. It was a beautiful place with majestic mountains and a mesmerizing lake, and it housed the Edgewood Tahoe Golf Course where the celebrity golf tournament would take place.

I was like a little kid as I talked with Bob about the tournament. It was obvious that I was more than eager to arrive, meet new people, and reconnect with old friends.

We hadn't been driving thirty minutes when the nausea unexpectedly hit me again, so much so that we had to stop at a hotel for the night. Fortunately, we had arrived a day early, so we had the wiggle room in Bob's schedule.

That evening, I couldn't eat dinner. All I could do was lie in bed.

In the middle of the night, I woke up unable to breathe. My chest got tighter and tighter as if an elephant was sitting on it. Placing my hand over my chest with one hand and shaking Bob from sleep with the other, I managed to say, "Bob, I can't breathe. I have to go to the hospital now."

He jumped up and quickly changed clothes. After helping me walk to the car, he drove me to the emergency room at Roseville Medical Center in Roseville, California. He explained to the receptionist that I just had my first chemotherapy treatment for breast cancer less than a week ago. The staff started working on me immediately. They were unbelievably wonderful.

A nurse checked my vitals and then strapped oxygen on my face. "Mrs. Kormondy, I'm not surprised you were having problems breathing. Your oxygen levels are low due to the high altitude here," she explained. "It's different than what you're used to. You're actually getting less oxygen with each breath."

She was right. The extra oxygen she gave me was like a lifeline, allowing me to breathe so much better.

After some IVs, a lot of tests, and several hours of treatment, a middle-aged doctor walked into my curtained-off "room" and examined me. He came up with the same conclusion. "So, you've probably been to this area of the country before and haven't had any problems breathing, right? Most people adjust fairly easily to the altitude change, but they didn't just have chemotherapy. You have, and with all that you've been through not even a week ago, your body wasn't able to make that adjustment to the decreased oxygen levels so well. That's why you felt like an elephant was sitting on your chest."

The doctor looked over at Bob and then back at me. His tone was very serious as he delivered his orders. "But when you get to Lake Tahoe, Mrs. Kormondy, you aren't going to be able to get out and about like usual, or else you're going to go through the same thing you did tonight. You're going to need to stay in your room and rest. Don't exert yourself. If you don't overdo and if you breathe slowly while you're here, your body should adjust to the high altitude."

His instructions and warning were quite a blow. I had looked forward to seeing the lake and watching the tournament like I had in previous years, not staying in my room.

He discharged me, and Bob and I went back to our hotel room.

The next morning, we finished our trip to Stateline and checked into our Tahoe resort. I was exhausted by then, but the view of the mountains and heavenly valley perked me up.

Bob made sure I was settled in and comfortable. He then had to leave to start the camera setup for the tournament. At the end of the day, he came back to the hotel, and I was rested up for dinner.

Then the next morning (and every morning for the rest of our trip), more hair was found on my pillow. I couldn't stand it. I would shake the hair off my pillowcase and turn it inside out until the housekeeper came to clean the room. I would ask her for clean pillowcases and apologize for all the hair on it. She was so kind and understanding.

Seeing the physical results of what cancer was doing to me was humbling. Of course, cancer wasn't making my hair fall out, but the weapon used against it was. If it wasn't for the cancer, then I wouldn't need that weapon, and I would still have all my hair.

These were the conversations and arguments I would have with myself. At the end, I would remind myself that there wasn't a thing I could do about it; I had no control over the matter. The only choice I had was to stop the chemo, but then again, that wouldn't end well for me.

So I would remind myself that I would rather be alive and bald than dead with my beautiful red hair. Still, the process was heart-wrenching, and the self-talk was not very successful.

Bob recognized how my hair loss affected my self-esteem, so when he was around me, he would give me reassuring glances and more hugs, telling me how beautiful I was. Those extra efforts on his part went a long way.

He loved me, balding head and all, but I wasn't sure the world was ready for it and would love me. So before we went out for dinner every evening, I would don a scarf or my new wig, and we would go somewhere to eat. It was actually the highlight of my day.

One night, however, I found myself unable to breathe again. Bob took me to the emergency room of a hospital about five minutes up the street. Now that we understood what was happening to me, we were able to cut through a lot of testing by the hospital. I was given oxygen for a couple of hours and then sent back to my hotel room.

During the day, I seemed to do better. However, I would be in that room, miserable . . . alone, bored, and wishing so much I could be there on the greens.

A person can only watch so much TV, so I filled my time with prayer and reading the Bible I had brought. Deep down, however, I knew I was too weak to watch the tournament in person. It's a lot of physical activity for the spectators as well the players because they all walk the golf course together, and those courses can be quite extensive in size.

This realization didn't take away from my disappointment of not being able to participate. After seeing how down I was about being confined to my room day after day, Bob took me to the lake and sat me down in one of the resort's Adirondack chairs so that I could look at its beauty.

While basking in its magnificence, one of Bob's friends walked over to us. "Hey, Bob, the crew's all down a bit farther on the beach. Why don't you and Evelyn join us?"

I looked at Bob with raised eyebrows. "Please, Bob. Can we?" I begged.

He studied me for a moment and then back at the direction from where his friend came. "Tell you what, Evie," he began, "I'll walk down there first to see how far it is. Then I'll come back. If it's not that far and I think you can make it, then we'll go."

Realizing I wasn't in any position to argue, I agreed to his suggestion. He left with his friend and was gone for a while. I stared at the scenery and basked in the peacefulness, thanking God for the opportunity to enjoy it all in person.

When Bob returned, he had another couple with him—a coworker named Christian Schwartzer and his wife.

Christian smiled as he approached me and clasped my hand. "I'm here for you, Evie," he said. He proceeded to pick me up like I was a ragdoll and carry me all the way down to the party, which was about the distance of two city blocks away, so that I could join everyone else.

I was a little bit embarrassed but appreciative. Bob would've carried me if his right arm hadn't been damaged from cancer.

People greeted me with such warmth and sincerity and treated me so kindly. Even though I was weak, I had a wonderful time.

When we got back to the hotel room, I was exhausted and ended up staying in my room and resting for the next two days with no further argument.

Then it was time to go home.

During the plane ride, I stared at my reflection in the window—solemn face framed by a scarf. I thought back over the past six days. It definitely wasn't the Lake Tahoe trip I had expected; it wasn't the Lake Tahoe trip I had experienced in previous years. Time for some introspection and being real and honest with myself.

Evelyn, I chided, *you've just entered this battle. Yes, you desperately wanted things to be normal, to be able to do what you've always done every time you went with Bob to the Tahoe tournament. You tuned out the logic as to why you shouldn't have come. You weren't thinking about your condition when you made the decision to come here. You had forgotten about the high altitude. You can't make rational decisions with chemo fog.*

Your life isn't what it was in those previous Lake Tahoe years. Taking this trip was not going to make everything normal again. You're being treated for cancer, Evie! Cancer! Accept it, and quit thinking you can mentally put away and ignore the physical. This trip proved that trying to force yourself to do what your body can't do isn't helping anyone, just the opposite. You have to be patient with yourself.

After my scolding and reality check, I made a mental note to stop making decisions during the chemo fog. I just wasn't going to be able to think everything through anymore, at least not until chemo was over. I finally got it. Normalcy didn't have a place in my life right now.

Staring out the plane window, I wondered if my life would ever be normal again.

−38−

Taking Back My Power

I continued to have so many other questions; one was my ability to fight this battle. The end seemed so far away.

But God knew my fears, even better than I did. So He sent me an angel that went by the name of Laurie Scott McSwain. She called out of the blue and introduced herself.

"Evelyn Kormondy?" a soft voice with a slightly fun lilt asked on the other end of the phone.

"Yes, this is Evelyn," I responded, somewhat skeptical.

"You don't know me," she started, "but my name's Laurie McSwain. We have a friend in common named Joe. He told me about you and your breast cancer fight from the very beginning of your diagnosis. I guess the reason he told me about you is that I know what you're going through. I've also gone through breast cancer. I had chemo and lost my hair. I also had a double mastectomy and radiation. I know how scary it can be, and unless you've been there yourself, it's hard for anyone else to understand. So, the reason for my call is to let you know that I'm here if you have any questions about any of it."

Oh my, did I have questions! And I needed to talk to someone who had been there, done that! The next thing I knew, Laurie and I were deep in a conversation, me the student and her the seasoned teacher and such a kind and patient one at that.

Over the next week, she called to see if I needed anything. "Evelyn, would you mind if I drop by your house in a couple of days? I would really like to meet you."

"I don't mind at all," I exclaimed. "In fact, I would love it!" We had such a connection.

Two days later, right on time, a red-headed woman stood on my front porch area holding a box. She must be Laurie!

As soon as I opened my door, she looked me over quickly. "Here," she extended the box in front of her with a warm and contagious smile. "I brought you a care package."

Excited to talk to her in person, I invited her in and took the box from her. I was like a kid on Christmas morning!

She stood next to me as I opened it. Inside was a wig, several scarves, an ice pack for the hot flashes I would soon be feeling, a book that answered more of my questions, and a bear with "Hugs" written across its chest. She thought of everything I would need during that time.

Her high energy level was infectious, and I enjoyed just being around her. Here she was, taking time with someone she had just met. Since then, we have had many conversations and developed a friendship.

Laurie didn't have breast cancer for a long time after her treatments ended. Then she got diagnosed with metastatic breast cancer and has been living with it for years. She's on medication, but she is enjoying life with her children, her father, and her granddaughter.

Even with everything she has and is going through, she's an unbelievable force in this world against breast cancer. She not only fights it herself, but she still helps others fight it as well. Every day, she's on Facebook educating people and sharing lessons about metastatic breast cancer.

Laurie McSwain is a hero, a leader in this battle for lives. I love her strength, her kindness, and her love for the world. Today, I am proud to call this amazing woman my dear friend.

Laurie's visit was just in time for my second chemo treatment on July 31. My attitude was now different as I approached it. The first treatment had broken me, had kicked me when I was down. As a result, I had gained respect for the drugs after feeling their power unleashed upon me.

That didn't mean I had given in and given up my fight, just that I knew the enemy better. So many things I didn't have control over, and I had to learn to pick my battles.

One was my hair. So much of it had fallen out over the past three weeks. Initially, seeing large clumps of it here, there, and everywhere devastated me. And as Bob told me before we left for Tahoe, there was nothing to be done to stop this effect. So I came to accept it, making scarves and the wig Nita had bought me part of my wardrobe.

As I got dressed to go to the Mercy infusion center, I decided to show off my new wig. When my friend Kathy McCoy picked me up, she loved it! Having her feedback meant a lot to me and boosted my confidence to go another round.

I had previously shared with her what had happened to me after the last treatment, so bless her heart, she had gone ahead and packed herself an overnight bag . . . just in case. Neither of us knew what to expect.

I walked into that same large room filled with recliners; IV poles; and wigs, scarves, or turbans on top of the occupants' heads. I felt as if I now fit in more with most of the other women there. My wig was my membership card to this special group, one that nobody wanted to belong to, but once involuntarily inducted into it, the unspoken camaraderie provided strength.

The nurse pointed to my assigned recliner. After sitting in it, I bared my upper chest portal without any prompting. Turned out, that port was a wonderful thing. Didn't feel a thing.

As the poison flooded through my body, I glanced around the room at each woman and studied them one by one. They seemed different to me now, each representing their own unique story. If ever given the chance, I would love to hear them because they all could teach me a thing or two. But in the meantime, we shared an unspoken request to respect the other's privacy. We understood this shared plight, regardless of where we were in it. We sat in silence and just accepted the poison and mentally prepared for its aftermath.

That night, the chemicals inside me raged, resulting in severe nausea. It was going to be another long one, so I decided to stay in the bathroom to let the drugs do to me what they desired, what they were going to do anyway.

Then as soon as I felt strong enough and fairly sure that there was nothing left in my stomach, I hobbled to my bed and crawled under the covers. Kathy placed an empty trash can next to it in case I couldn't make it to the bathroom in time should I be assaulted again.

The next day, weakness racked my body. At times, I could barely pray, but God knew my requests. Then I started sniffling and sneezing.

I thought, *Gosh, my immune system is so bad that I caught a cold.*

Fortunately, the symptoms weren't bad enough to call the doctor. Plus, I was sure that once I began to build my strength back up after that last round of chemo, they would go away.

And as if all that wasn't difficult enough, I kept finding massive amounts of my hair on my pillow. Tired of going through that every day, I evaluated the situation.

Well, Evelyn, I thought, *you've got more bald spots than hair. You've been picking up hair from the floor, the counter, your pillow, and it's become quite a depressing chore. It's just gotten to be too much. It's all going to fall out here soon anyway, so you might as well end the long and drawn-out torture of waiting for the inevitable.*

I made the decision to take back my power. Bob was out of town, so I called my father.

"Daddy, would you take me to your barber? I want to get my head shaved so I don't have to see my hair laying around everywhere anymore."

I would have loved to have asked my mother, but we hadn't told her about my cancer because she was battling arterial disease. We hated keeping this from her because I could have used her nurturing and pulled from her strength. If she wasn't so sick, I was certain she would have been able to handle it. But she had already lost one daughter to breast cancer and almost lost another. She had seen what we had been through with Bob's cancer. We just didn't want to burden her with this additional stressor.

After a few moments of silence on the other end, my dad agreed to take me to his barber. He picked me up a couple of hours later.

We walked into the shop together. Then he grabbed my hand and held it as I told his barber what I wanted him to do. "Please, just go ahead and shave the rest of it off."

I removed my scarf, and the barber studied my head and nodded with no emotion, only acknowledgement. He pointed to the chair next to him. "You can sit here."

We all watched in the mirror as he took his electric clippers to my scalp. It was like a horror show, where you know you should look away, but you simply can't. So, I watched every stroke he made on my scalp as the tufts of red hair fell to the ground.

Then it was over. The person in the mirror was somebody else; at least it appeared that way. Having a bald head was strange. Out of the corner of my eye, I could see my dad tearing up when he saw me in the mirror. He quickly looked away when he realized I was watching him.

It had to be hard for him to see how sick his little girl was. His baby had her head shaven because of the very same thing that had already brought massive devastation and loss to his family.

After a few minutes, he brought his eyes back to the mirror. The three of us stared pensively at my reflection in silence.

Dad forced a smile on his face and blurted, "Evelyn, all these years and I never knew you had the perfect-shaped head for baldness." His light-hearted remark broke through the heavy atmosphere.

We all enjoyed a good laugh, I think mostly in relief from taking our minds off of what my shaved scalp front and center represented. By the time we left the shop, I walked to our car holding my bald head high!

Over the next couple of days, I found out that others shared the same sentiments as my dad. My beautiful daughters would say, "You are rockin' the bald look,

Evelyn. Just put on a pair of big-hoop earrings, a smile, and voila! You're gorgeous!"

Most importantly was what Bob thought. When he first saw me after my barber visit, a big smile emerged on his face. "Evie, you look really good with a bald head."

I sensed his sincerity and gave him a big hug of appreciation. Then I told him about the experience and how hard it was to sit in that barber chair knowing all my hair would be gone.

"There was no hope in keeping it," I added.

Bob's eyes stayed fixed on my head, and his smile didn't waver. "I'm proud of you. To give up your hair to save your existence is not a bad trade."

He always knew what to say and what I needed to hear. So I happily and joyfully sported my bald head for the rest of the world to see.

– 3 9 –

Pink Tears

As time went on, I started building up a nice collection of wigs and beautiful scarves to stylishly cover up my head. However, one of many unpleasant side effects from chemo was the intense hot flashes. They caused a heat inside my body that made me feel as if I was on fire. My whole body and head would sweat and soak the scarf.

Bob observed my challenges one day and suggested, "Evie, when you're hot, just go bald-headed. You look beautiful without anything on your head anyway."

Between his encouragement and my bullheadedness, I shed the scarves and wigs about 40 percent of the time, usually when I was home or in the neighborhood, and then walked around proudly. I was going to prove to cancer that it was not going to control every aspect of my life. But there were times when I simply wanted to "accessorize" my attire, and a wig or scarf made a great fashion statement. Strange how my perspective had changed from the first day I saw a large amount of hair on my pillow.

By the time I had my third chemotherapy treatment on August 28, 2013, I felt like a veteran. Everything became routine. Do this, then do that, and then do this and that.

Part of the routine, unfortunately, was the aftermath that consisted of extreme nausea. It would wallop me and force me to stay close to, if not in, the bathroom throughout the night.

I reminded myself, *You're halfway there, Evelyn. Three treatments down and three to go. You can do it, girl!*

Fortunately, the day after this latest treatment, I had gained some strength despite the previous night, which was great. Bob was due to come home, and I would be able to enjoy him much more.

A few minutes before he was supposed to arrive, I sat and waited in the family room with one eye on the television and one on the clock. Then right on time, I heard the door close behind him. I was so happy, especially as I watched him walking quickly to me.

He wrapped his arms around me. Now I was back to being safe and knew all would be okay. The overwhelming emotions bubbling up inside caused me to cry.

After a few moments, Bob pulled back.

I blurted out, "I missed you so much, Bob! I'm so glad you're home."

His eyes searched my face with an expression of both concern and love. "Evie, your tears are pink," he commented.

Confused, I wiped my tears off my face with the back of my ring finger. Looking down at my hand, the tears did appear to have a pink tinge. The curiosity motivated me to stand and walk to the bathroom mirror where I was shocked to see that my tears were indeed pink. Bob followed behind me.

Staring at my reflection, I said, "I guess they put so much of that red 'angel of healing' into my body that it has to come out some way. Apparently, it's mixing with my tears and turning them pink."

Bob looked at me with his eyebrows furrowed. "Red angel of healing?" he asked.

"That's right," I responded. "I refuse to give that red devil anymore credit and power, so I call it God's angel of healing that's getting the bad stuff out of my body."

Bob nodded in understanding. "Well, I love your pink tears." He then gave me a kiss on the top of my head. "I'm going to put my bags in the bedroom. What time do we need to go back to the hospital for your IV and shot?"

That put a real damper on the moment. "Three. I wished I didn't have to go back to the hospital at all," I added.

"I know, I know," Bob agreed. "But you always say that, and then afterward, you always admit how much better you feel because of it. Hey, I'm going to be with you for this one."

His words energized me. Whatever I had to do, I always felt much more relaxed when he was by my side. When he was home and I was being given some type of treatment, he would sit in a tiny chair next to my big comfortable one. Not for one moment did I believe he was comfortable, but he didn't care. He was determined to be there with me. It didn't matter if we watched TV or just talked, he would hold my hand and rub it to make me feel better.

So I always tried to schedule my treatments on the days I knew he would be home. Having him with me made them much less stressful and lonely as opposed to those treatments when a friend or family member dropped me off and picked me up from them.

As soon as we were back home again, Bob continued to treat me with such kindness and gentleness, waiting on me to make sure I had what I needed. Our roles had reversed from over eighteen months ago, and he was now the caretaker and I the patient. Fortunately, he didn't have to give me IVs or pour Ensure into a feeding tube, and his chemo treatments were not as powerful as mine. It was hard on him nevertheless, especially when he had to leave me to go out of town.

He also took his role as the breadwinner seriously. So he was torn between financially supporting us and physically and emotionally supporting me with his presence. I would reassure him every time and remind him that I had a whole support team when he wasn't around consisting of family, friends, and other church members. Someone was always with me if I needed them.

But having someone with me was not always in my best interest. With chemo compromising the immune system, sometimes my support team could only support me from afar. And it could be very lonely.

For instance, when my cold wouldn't go away, and I began coughing as if something was caught in my lungs, Bob took me to see the doctor. I was diagnosed with pneumonia and hospitalized for three days. Bob was the only one allowed to visit with me, but he could only come at night. I hated to be by myself. Even though I was sick, I would have loved to have my support team with me. Thankfully, though, I could see my husband.

Bob and I enjoyed being together, even when one of us was sick. Time always flew. Then before we both knew it, he was off again. I rested a lot, and his absence gave me the opportunity to talk with friends and family. Those conversations deepened bonds that may not have happened otherwise, a great example of God's promises given in Romans 8:28: "And we know that in all things God works for the good of those who love him, who have been called according to his purpose (NIV)."

Then on September 17, I had another chemo treatment.

Four down, two to go.

−40−

The Intensity Intensifies

I braced myself for what was sure to come that night, knowing that tomorrow would be better. For the first three treatments, I had managed to get through and beyond them with the worst of the sickness occurring soon afterwards. Then I would gain strength with each new day.

Of course, the chemo fog remained, but I was getting used to that too. I figured it would hang around as long as I was having treatments.

The night after this fourth treatment, however, was more intense than ever before. I had never been sick to this extreme. The nausea and what accompanied it were so bad that I truly felt as if I were dying at that time. Even the IV for dehydration and nausea shot given to me the next day did nothing to improve my situation.

Regardless of my prayers for healing, the sickness engulfed me. It didn't only affect my body but my mind as well. Things started to seem dismal, and I had a deep feeling that I wasn't going to survive. At least if I did die, I would be going to my heavenly home and be with my Heavenly Father and my family members who were already there. Still, I didn't want to die; I wanted to be here for my large and beautiful family.

Unlike past treatments, the next morning didn't get better either. Then every day thereafter, there was no letting up as depression refused to relinquish its hold. It didn't matter how foggy my brain was or how sick I felt, if I wanted to push past the physical, I knew I didn't have a choice but to engage with my mind. I tried my best to hold on, but honestly, there were some really bad times that made me wonder just how long I could.

If I wasn't going to be healed, I prayed for Bob's healing to stay with him. I loved him so much.

With no end in sight, it looked as if I may lose this battle. If that happened, I wanted my family members to know what they meant to me. So I pushed myself to compose letters to my husband, my children, my parents, and the rest of my wonderful family, each one personal. At the end, I would pronounce a blessing over them.

I was too weak to handwrite them, so I used a headset microphone for my computer and spoke my thoughts and feelings into it. My audible words would then be converted into writing.

Even at that, I could only do about a letter a day because it was so emotionally draining; I wanted them to understand just how much I loved them. The thought of not being a part of their future, not being able to see them grow up, was almost more than I could take. They loved me, but I wanted to make sure they realized what an amazing difference they had made in my life by being part of it. Then I would print them out, sign them, and add little hearts, kisses, and a smiley face.

To intensify my sickness and gloom-and-doom emotions, I felt like every one of my bones were being broken one by one. Thank God Bob was with me at the time because never had I endured such severe and relentless pain that not only attacked my bones but also my nerves and really, everything. It hurt so bad, I just wanted it to stop. I prayed for it to stop; I begged for it to stop. I asked Bob why it wouldn't stop!

In an effort to describe the pain, I would say it felt like a little man was inside my body with a hammer and was unmercifully pounding away with it on different joints, like my kneecaps, ankles, and elbows.

With almost every breath, I continued praying and crying out to God. Bob also prayed with me. We knew that God was the answer. We had witnessed, observed, and experienced Him coming through for us too many times to believe differently.

Then as the saying goes—"This too shall end"— and so it went with this indescribably harsh illness and body pains. I lived to tell the story, not to murmur and complain and depict myself as a victim; I don't want to scare anyone about the side effects of chemo. The purpose of telling you about what happened to me is to provide encouragement to those who will be or are taking chemo. It's to testify to the fact that you will survive and that this too shall pass; God will help you. You too will have your own story to tell about surviving cancer so that you can inspire others.

After several weeks, I started regaining some strength and thanked God for the faithfulness He demonstrated time and again. As difficult and challenging as Bob's cancer treatments were, it had grown my faith exponentially. Then when I was faced with my own cancer, my foundation and trust in God were sturdy and didn't, would *not* falter. I came out of it even stronger.

One day, the devil's going to learn that when you come after the Kormondys, it's only increasing our reliance and faith in God!

But the enemy will test your faith. The night of my fifth treatment on October 8 was difficult but nothing compared to the aftermath of the last treatment.

The next day, I felt bad, but I was scheduled for my IV and shot. This time around, I believed they would improve my situation like they did after the first three treatments. The previous one, well, that turned out to be the exception to the rule, and I prayed it would remain that way and not be repeated.

While in the area, I went to my appointment with Dr. Stevens first. But this wasn't just any appointment. This time we were going to talk about getting me on the schedule for my double mastectomy so that they could finally cut this nasty cancer out of me, even though it meant removing both of my breasts. Consequently, I approached this visit with equal amounts of eagerness and trepidation.

Dr. Stevens needed to make sure I still wanted to have both breasts removed as opposed to only the one with the tumor. As a woman, it was hard to say, "Take them both."

I mean, what would I look like without my breasts? Would I be changed, not just physically on the outside but on the inside as well? Would I feel like less of a woman? Would others perceive me that way?

What would I look like with reconstruction surgery, that is, *IF* I went through reconstruction surgery? At this point in time, the thought of having to go through one more medical procedure wasn't anything I really wanted to do, especially if I didn't really have to.

Bob held my hand during the entire visit. It didn't matter to him if I had breasts or not; he only saw me as beautiful. He only wanted me alive and with him. His unconditional love helped me to make the final decision—to give up my symbol of femininity for the greater good.

Women should never have to question their femininity. It isn't about breasts and ovaries but about their God-given soul. My decision had come down to recognizing how both of my breasts had become the enemy in this war. My family history was proof of that. Even though only one of my breasts seemed to be trying to kill me now, if I didn't have the other one removed as well, it would more than likely try to kill me sooner or later. No, thank you. They were both lethal, so they both had to go. I really had no other choice but to have the double mastectomy.

Bob drove me to Dr. Stevens's office. I stared out the passenger window for most of the trip there. It was going to be a warm day, yet everything about that day seemed cold. Basically, I was going to see her to discuss what felt like euthanasia to me. We needed to kill my breasts before they killed me.

During the appointment, I assured her that I had not changed my mind; I wanted to increase my odds of survival because I wanted to live for my husband, my children, and the rest of my family and friends. For me, it was a no-brainer, especially after two sisters had to battle this same cancer.

With my decision recorded, our questions were now focused on the surgery itself, from everything that it would entail before, during, and after, to the recovery time and all that I would go through.

Dr. Stevens shared a wealth of information with us. I tried so hard to grasp it all, but the brain fog prevented me from comprehending it clearly. Thank God, Bob was with me. I truly would not have been able to handle this discussion without his presence, support, and understanding of what she relayed to us.

He stepped in and patiently discussed things with me so that I could better understand what was about to happen to me.

– 41 –

You Are Stronger than Cancer

The next day, October 10, Bob took me to see the plastic surgeon, Dr. Paine. I had met him during my tour at Cox Breast Clinic, and I had liked him. His confidence was contagious.

Although reconstructive surgery still seemed so far away, my medical team encouraged me to see the plastic surgeon before the mastectomy. Both surgeons worked in tandem with each other. My decisions of what I wanted for my reconstructed breasts could help Dr. Stevens when she did the mastectomy. Consequently, both surgeons coordinating their efforts would give me the best outcome in the reconstruction. It also gave me hope, something to look forward to, a benchmark that represented healing and the end of this journey and the start of reconstructing my life.

When we arrived, Dr. Paine's waiting room was packed with other patients vying for his attention and expertise. After waiting for longer than I wanted, a nurse finally called us back.

I still wasn't sold on going through a major surgery to get new breasts, but I had already made the appointment. Since Bob was with me, I thought I might as well go through with it, see what the doctor had to say.

Dr. Paine explained that after the double mastectomy, he would insert expanders under the skin where the breasts are now. They would prepare my body for the reconstruction of the skin that would be left behind from the mastectomy. Then over a period of six weeks prior to the surgery, he would be injecting a saline solution into the expanders to stretch out the skin for the implants.

It sounded painful. "Will it hurt?" I asked.

He shrugged. "You may feel some discomfort. As the expanders get larger, the area will feel tighter."

Dr. Paine showed me actual implants so that I could see the differences between them. "Here," he said as he handed them to me. "Go ahead and touch them and see how they feel and how heavy each is."

"What are other differences?" I asked. "Is one safer than the other?"

He assured me that both were safe, but both did have some risks. "Saline implants are filled with sterile saline water," he responded, "and silicone implants are filled with silicone gel."

"What happens if one leaks or ruptures?" I asked as I continued holding the implants in my hands and evaluating them.

He shrugged. "Let's hope that doesn't happen, but if it does, then they can be fixed. With the saline implant, you'll need to have it removed and replaced. With the silicone implant, you may not even know it's ruptured, but if it goes on too long without being addressed, you may start feeling some pain. We would need to do an MRI to see what's going on with it."

I ended up choosing the saline implant. They simply sounded safer. I didn't like the idea of silicone gel running wild and free in my body if an implant leaked or ruptured. On the other hand, if a saline bag leaked or ruptured, then sterile saline water would invade my body. That sounded much more appealing.

"Okay," he said and noted my answer. "Saline it is. Would you prefer a round look or teardrop look?"

I glanced back and forth between Bob and Dr.

Paine in confusion, hoping to find some clue to help me understand this question. Bob's eyes had widened, and he shrugged as in "I don't know what to tell you."

Turning back to the doctor, I asked, "What's the difference? All I know is that I want them to look exactly like they do now, you know, the same shape but smaller—a B-cup—and without the cancer."

His eyebrows furrowed in the middle, and now, he was the one looking confused. "Why a B-cup?"

"Well, I've been a double D since I was fifteen years old," I explained. "I don't want to be that large again. It can be uncomfortable, and I want comfort, so I really would prefer a B-cup."

He shook his head. "You don't want to be a B-cup, Evelyn. That's like not having any breasts at all. Women come in here wanting to be a D-cup."

We debated B-cup versus D-cup. Eventually, he convinced me to go with a small C-cup.

He gave me a binder with pictures of breasts he had done. "Here, look through these pictures and see if you can find one that you like."

I opened the book and studied each picture before coming across the perfect one for me. "There," I pointed to the picture, "that's what I want."

Dr. Paine pursed his lips. "We can't make them look exactly like that, Evelyn. That one isn't going to work with your body."

Well, he was the expert, so if he said it wasn't going to work with my body, then there must be a good reason. Still, it was disappointing, and I was now even more confused than before.

With so many questions, glaring brain fog, and so many important decisions to make, I became overwhelmed. What if I made the wrong decision because I couldn't think everything through?

I glanced at Bob with tears in my eyes. He would be able to tell me what to do if the model I wanted wasn't going to work.

He smiled, his eyes revealing love and support. "Sweetheart, it doesn't even matter if you do this reconstruction surgery. You're beautiful just the way you are, and you'll be more beautiful after the mastectomy, with or without breasts."

Then he put his attention onto Dr. Paine. "Doctor, just put one in each hand for me. Let me see what they feel like." He then chuckled. He obviously was trying to make me laugh because the atmosphere in the room had gotten so heavy.

It worked. I laughed so hard I had tears running down my cheeks.

Bob deliberated between both implants, weighing each one. "I think the round one looks more like Evie." He placed his eyes on me. "Honey, do you want these round ones? They remind me of you."

Again, I broke down and couldn't stop laughing. "Sure, honey, they'll be fine."

Bob was wonderful at taking the pressure off me and making me laugh at a difficult situation.

That appointment with Dr. Paine turned out to be very productive. We had accomplished several things, including choosing the type of implants and the size. We even scheduled our next appointment for the following week. In the meantime, he would be consulting with Dr. Stevens about my decisions. Then we would be able to firm everything up the next time I saw him.

Bob and I walked out of his office holding hands. We discussed our choices that night to make sure we were happy with them. Admittedly, I was excited and full of hope about this next phase of my life.

I believe that hope empowered me. Even though it had been only four days since my fifth chemo treatment, it gave me strength so that Bob and I could attend the Victory in Pink event for those who have or had breast cancer. It was held at the St. Johns Town Center.

Earlier in the week, a friend had recommended me to the gentleman putting on a show at the event. We spoke, and he asked me to be a model for it, which was basically me modeling myself and how well I was doing so that I could encourage others.

He said, "Rebecca Thomas from the evening news will introduce you. Then you'll walk out on a long stage and read something positive that you've written. That's all there is to it."

Sounded simple enough, so I agreed to do it.

Victory in Pink ended up having a tremendous turnout. Bob and I walked around and talked with other cancer survivors as well as doctors. The event had tattoo artists to cover our physical scars. Everyone was given a T-shirt on which to write a meaningful phrase. Mine was "Day by day," my motto, because it described how I dealt with cancer.

When the time for the show started approaching, I walked over to the big stage to register. I told those to whom I gave my paperwork about Bob and his cancer.

One of the ladies said, "You and Bob have to walk the runway together!"

I wasn't sure Bob wanted to walk the runway, but he did it for me. So we stood in line until they called our names.

When Rebecca introduced both of us, she then proceeded to tell the audience about my cancer as I walked out. The crowd cheered.

She said, "If you're wondering why Bob is here on the stage with Evelyn, well, Bob is also a cancer survivor."

The crowd went crazy. The whole experience was overwhelming and exhilarating, and we were having fun with it. Bob twirled me across the stage.

Then Rebecca read a quote from us that said, "You are stronger than the cancer. Let me repeat—you are stronger than the cancer!"

Bob kissed me, and we glided off the stage.

−42−

Team Kormondy

Love is a wonderful and powerful thing to feel and know when going through cancer. From it spurs patience and understanding.

My mind still wasn't operating at optimal level, so Bob stepped in to fill the gap and remained super-focused on my care. He managed to get through each obstacle, whether it was routine or unexpected.

On top of helping me, he also had his own medical appointments he had to attend, at least monthly, with either his surgeon, his oncologist, or his radiation oncologist. I couldn't go with him anymore since I was too weak from my own fight. Plus, we knew in our hearts that he was clear of any cancer. To us, these appointments were merely routine.

Whether we were battling Bob's cancer or my own, we would not have successfully gotten through any of it if not for our support team of family and friends, including those from our Sunday school class. They prayed for us and brought by much-appreciated meals. Their outpouring of love was crucial in so many ways and on so many levels.

We truly enjoyed when they came by and visited. However, during those times when either Bob's or my immune system was compromised, visitors were limited to few. My parents were part of those few, which made seeing them a bigger treat. But my mother's arteries were clogging up faster than the doctors could help her. Because it affected her brain, my dad needed to be at home with her. So during those times when I felt stronger, we would visit them.

With my double mastectomy right around the corner, I wanted to visit my mother. I wasn't feeling quite as strong as I would like, but seeing her beforehand was very important to me. No matter what she was suffering through, her demeanor never changed. She remained the kindest woman I've ever known. I needed my mother's love right now. Simply being in her presence was a huge support for me.

Bob understood. He didn't have any family around. Both parents had passed, and his two brothers lived out of town. So he encouraged me to spend time with my mother as much as possible.

The morning of our planned visit, I was so excited and considered it a big treat. Nevertheless, I still didn't want her to know that I was sick. So I changed out of something loose that I wore around the house and put on a cute dress. Looking in the mirror, I still looked sick. So I applied a little makeup to my pale face and put on a wig.

I looked in the mirror one last time. Much improved. Dressing up like this actually made me feel better, even though it exhausted me.

Bob then drove me the seven miles to my parents' house.

I was unable to be my usual energetic self, and I knew she would pick up on that and wonder. So I went ahead and told her I had a stomachache and wasn't feeling well that day, which was the truth. During that time and most days, I never felt well and did struggle with stomachaches.

She and I sat on the couch together and talked, but she wasn't remembering a whole lot. That never kept her from wearing that big smile on her face and giving a big hug to everyone in her path. It didn't matter if it was her family at home or those at church as Dad pushed her in her wheelchair. Everyone loved my mother, and I mean *everyone*. She was an amazing woman!

Arterial disease couldn't steal her wisdom and discernment, though. At one point during our conversation, she stared at my head with a confused look. She leaned over toward me and stroked my hair, my wig. She had to have known it wasn't real; after all, I was her daughter.

Trying to not upset her, I said, "Mom, we're playing dress-up today. Do you like my wig?"

She smiled and nodded. "Yes, I do."

I grabbed her hand and held it. Her smile of understanding caused a tear to well up in one of her eyes. She then pulled off my wig.

My eyes started to tear up as I realized we weren't fooling her in the least bit. She knew. We didn't tell her, but she knew.

Mom patted my hand. She then leaned in closer and whispered, "Evelyn, you know sometimes, it's okay to cry. I love you."

I nodded, but I was unsuccessful at trying to hold it together. The tears were determined to flow.

And as my mother and I stared into each other's eyes, I didn't care anymore. I needed my mom, and deep within me, I knew she needed her daughter.

In that moment, our bond deepened. We understood each other, and I sensed that we were both okay.

−43−

Preparing to Face the Giant

Toward the middle of October, the mental and physical preparations for the surgery ramped up. It would not be the final battle, but it was the event we had all been waiting for. It was the event that would remove that nasty tumor once and for all.

The mastectomy was scheduled after the fifth chemotherapy treatment because typically, the sixth was more of a precaution. By then, the tumors would have shrunk as much as they were going to shrink. So the next step would be to cut out all the cancer they could get (if not all of it) via the surgery.

Sure, my body was still beat up from the last treatment, but it didn't matter. The medical team just kept going at the cancer because they knew that the cancer was going to keep going at me. They didn't let my body rest because the cancer didn't rest.

So it was go, go, go on this ride and realize that

you will be okay when it finally comes to a stop. God knew you when He knitted you in your mother's womb (Psalm 139:13), and together, you are writing your story all along the way.

Bob decided not to accept any jobs until December 22, which would be a Jaguars home game, so that he wouldn't have to leave me. Fortunately, it was the slow time of the year for golf, so this football game was great timing. Not only did it give him the chance to work in town, but we also both loved the Jaguars!

Emotionally, I needed him with me on so many levels. Major surgery was about to take place on my body, and you bet I was scared! But when I was with Bob . . . he had a way of making me feel as if I could slay giants.

About ten days prior to the scheduled surgery, he took me to Mercy for pre-op tests, such as blood work, PET scan, MRI, CAT scan, and an ultrasound. Then the week before the surgery, it was time to meet with Dr. Stevens for a pre-op appointment. She shared my test results with me.

"Great news, Evelyn!" she started as she scanned the reports, "the chemo worked; your tumor has shrunk. The smaller size is going to make the surgery easier and increase our chances of catching everything." She wore a big smile when she turned to look at me.

She was right; that was great news! All those times of getting so sick had paid off. It was all worth it.

Dr. Stevens then explained everything she would be doing in the surgery. She also informed me about what would happen afterward, such as the pain I would experience and the post-op care I would require, especially with the drains.

Bob and I glanced at each other in confusion.

"Drains?" I asked.

"Yes. We'll be inserting tubes that are each about fourteen to eighteen inches long into your chest to drain the blood from the surgery. At the other end of these tubes are bulbs that will collect the blood. The amount of blood will then need to be measured several times a day. Once there's no more blood, we can remove the drains."

"Will the drains hurt, Dr. Stevens?" I asked. I was already dreading this surgery, and these "drains" increased my anxiety.

"Oh no. They don't hurt at all," she responded.

We went home and discussed what she told us and

nailed down the details. We talked about the post-op care, including the drains.

Then we addressed my biggest fear, even bigger than the surgery itself—me without breasts and what I would look like. I still had concerns as to whether I would still feel like a woman. For many years after my hysterectomy in my twenties, I felt so inadequate. My female reproductive system had been removed, leaving me unable to have any babies.

Now, this cancer had taken my long red hair. And soon, the doctor would be removing what I perceived to be my last remaining body part that would identify me as a feminine, sexy, and pretty woman.

My husband again reassured me that I was concerned over something that didn't bother him in the least bit. "I love you, Evie. Your life is more important to me than your breasts. I would rather have you alive without breasts than buried with them. I want us to have a wonderful life together regardless. And if you decide not to have reconstruction surgery, I'll tell you again what I've been telling you—I'll still love you. I'll love you either way."

Yes, I had heard Bob tell me all this before, and his

words were appreciated each time. Still, I don't think I could hear them enough. Removing my breasts was a really big deal, and my insecurities kept cropping up. I guess I needed to know he hadn't changed his mind even though deep down, I was pretty sure he hadn't.

This time around, however, I listened to his words; I mean I *really* listened. They strengthened and empowered me as they took root inside my heart.

Contentment and confidence replaced insecurity and fear. I had Bob's blessing to get rid of my breasts; I had his support, even his encouragement. Now I was ready for surgery.

The day before, however, I was given a radioactive shot, also called radiation therapy, in my port. It's given to some people to target cancer cells that remain after the chemo.

I couldn't help but have some fun with the name "radiation." I asked the medical staff questions, such as "Will this shot cause me to glow?" "Do you think I should now support nuclear power since I am nuclear power?"

Despite my joking, in the back of my mind, I was concerned about how it would affect me. So I had to remind myself that it was supposed to do really good things for me, and at this point, I needed really good things that would get rid of whatever cancer insisted on plaguing me.

Then the day of the surgery finally arrived.

Bob woke up smiling as always and gave me a big hug. We lay together in bed for a few minutes before he got up to start the coffee, and I took a shower.

While the water heated up, I looked at my breasts in the mirror, realizing that in a few hours, I would never see them again. I then stepped into the shower and touched my breasts, realizing that I would never feel them again.

Tears fell from my eyes and mixed with the shower water. It was heart-wrenching to think that part of my body, part of me was going to be taken away from me forever.

Why did I get cancer? Why does anyone get cancer? I didn't know whether I would ever get the answers to these questions.

The surgical center had called the day before, reminding me to wear loose-fitting clothes. Since I would be wearing the same clothes to and from the hospital, they suggested my shirt have buttons down the front so that I could easily access the bandages once I came home.

Their words played in front of me like a mirage. Bandages in the front . . . bandages to cover the area where my breasts had once been. More tears flowed from my eyes as I visualized what that would look like.

By the time I walked into the kitchen, I was sniffling.

Bob stopped and watched me a moment before coming over to give me a big hug. "Honey, it's going to be okay. You are what's most important."

I allowed myself to linger in his arms before I finished getting ready. Just like it was when we left the house for Bob's surgery, which now seemed like a lifetime ago, it was dark outside because we had to check into the surgical center at 6 a.m.

Our mood and emotions during the drive were up and down—we were happy and relieved to get this over with soon, and we were scared, at least I was, wondering what the aftermath would bring.

Our conversations dwindled off, and I sat in silence. I couldn't help but question whether or not I had the strength to get through it. I had yet to fully recuperate from everything that had happened thus far, and the chemo treatments had completely drained and exhausted me.

Before I knew it, we were pulling into the parking lot, arriving in plenty of time. Sitting in the waiting room was agonizing. I just wanted this over and done!

But then moments before I went into surgery, Bob, my dad, and my pastor were all with me, praying over me and telling me that they loved me.

Bob said, "Evie, it's okay. I'll be here for you when you wake up."

Then my pastor prayed that the doctors would get all the cancer, and I would be cancer free in just a couple of hours.

These three men, each of them playing major roles in my life, gave me the courage to go to sleep knowing that I would wake up transformed!

– 44 –

We've Got This!

"Mrs. Kormondy? Mrs. Kormondy?"

The sound of a strange voice forced me to flicker open my eyes and push through the grogginess that shrouded my brain. I glanced around the unfamiliar setting. Mostly white. Beeping close by and others farther away. Antiseptic smell.

Huh?

Then it hit me. Oh, yes. I was in the hospital. I just had surgery. Thank God, I wasn't nauseous and vomiting like I had after my past surgery for cancer about fifteen years ago. I had been so afraid of that happening again, but this time, I had only a little nausea.

My eyes then fell onto a woman wearing blue scrubs. She was noting my vitals from the machine next to my bed. Then she looked down at me.

"Well, hello Mrs. Kormondy," she said with a smile. "I'm Carol. I'll be your nurse while you're in the recovery room. You just had surgery. Can I get you something?"

"I want Bob," I muttered. "Please, go get Bob."

"Okay. We'll get Bob in just a few minutes. We have to get you awake first, sweetheart."

I was motivated for her to get Bob, so I pushed myself through the grogginess of the remaining anesthesia. But the more awake I became, the more aware I became of the pain in my chest. It hurt so much, I could hardly catch my breath.

I said, "Oh dear. It hurts so bad. Why does it hurt so bad? I know surgery hurts; I just didn't think it would hurt this much. Please, can I have something for pain?"

"Of course, Mrs. Kormondy. I'll give you something right now." She took a syringe from the counter and proceeded to add it to my IV.

"Please get Bob," I repeated.

"Yes ma'am." She left, and the pain medication started to kick in some.

My hands moved slowly to my chest and paused before touching it. Once I did, tears welled up. What was once voluptuous was now flat like a boy's chest. They were gone . . . my breasts were gone! In their place were bandages wrapped completely around my upper torso. Tubes protruded through the gauze and then down to bulbs on the end. These must be what Dr. Stevens had told us about, the drains that would capture the blood from my chest.

Grief overwhelmed me, and I started crying for my loss. Then I saw Bob enter my small recovery area. He rushed over to me and sat next to me on the bed. I laid my head against his chest, and he gently cradled me in his arms, careful not to touch the front of my torso, until I stopped crying. Then we prayed.

"Evie," he said, "I know this may be hard to understand right now, but God has a reason for everything. He knows our plans in life. Remember Jeremiah 29:11—'For I know the plans I have for you," declares the LORD, "plans to prosper you and not to harm you, plans to give you hope and a future" (NIV). He will use this for His good. Losing your breasts wasn't in vain. When they took your breasts, they took the cancer with them."

I nodded in agreement and could now take a deep breath. He was my reason for living on this earth. I could not fight this battle without him. It was so wonderful to have him holding me even though I was in pain.

Eventually, I was transferred to a private room for a couple of days, and Bob stayed with me the whole time. The nurses showed him how to administer my medications for pain and infection as well as how to empty my drains into a measuring cup, write down the amount of blood in them, and then keep an eye on the drains for when they filled up again.

It was a lot of instructions at first, not to mention scary for me and probably somewhat scarier for Bob. The medical staff stressed that I need not fret over this uphill battle. I could take it day by day as the drainage slowed down more and more. At that point, the drains could be removed, which meant my body was in healing mode.

Day by day . . . Okay, Evelyn, this too shall end. Just accept it as part of the journey, and follow doctor's orders.

In my head, I started humming my anthem "Day by Day." I didn't need to hear the song playing; by now, I knew it by heart. Every time it played in my mind, I would just sing along with it there.

The words in this song gave me strength: "Day by day, oh dear Lord, three things I pray: To see Thee more clearly, love Thee more dearly, follow Thee more nearly day by day."

These words repeated themselves even while being pushed in a wheelchair to our car for Bob to take me home after being discharged on October 27. Once there, Bob helped me to the bathroom where I was finally in front of a mirror large enough to perform a self-assessment. I had just gotten comfortable with the no-hair look, but now, I was also going to have to contend with the no-breasts look. However, this loss was much more devastating than the loss of my hair.

Staring at myself, seeing the new me for the first time, I wondered, *Where am I? Where's Evelyn? I've lost me. Will I ever be able to find myself again?*

I broke down and cried, and Bob was right there behind me, wrapping his arms around my waist, telling me how beautiful I was. "Your hair will grow back, and if you want, there's always surgery for a new chest . . . just the way you want it." He smiled.

He loved me, hair or no hair, breasts or no breasts. His unconditional love reminded me that if he could love me like I was, then I needed to love me like I was too.

I walked into the family room and glanced around. Bob got busy laying out my medications as I sat down on our loveseat. We were on our own now—no nurses, no doctors, and no other medical staff to run to our aid should something go wrong.

"Bob," I said, "I'm going to sleep here on this loveseat. I think it's going to be too painful to lie down in our bed, not to mention the challenges we'd have with the drains and everything. And I can watch TV here, and when family visits, I'm already on my perch to resume my position as the quintessential hostess." I smiled.

"And I can sleep next to you," he offered.

Undoubtedly, he would have been more comfortable in the bed, but he didn't want to leave me out here alone. I recognized the sacrifice he was making overall, although I didn't think he looked at it that way.

In addition to the bed, he gave up the time he would normally be engaged in sports so that he could stay with me. Consequently, instead of spending our time together at the beach windsurfing, we were spending our time in our family room getting me through my recovery process.

It didn't take long for Bob to catch onto the whole post-op routine, including the drains. At least three times a day, he was right there doing a job that could not have been pleasant.

But we tried to make the best of it. I even got a special shirt from the American Cancer Society that had pockets to hold the drains. When I wanted to take a shower, Bob would put a lanyard around my neck beforehand and pin the drains to it.

Then no sooner had we adjusted to our new-yet-temporary norm of post-op recovery, I had to go back to Mercy to take my sixth and final chemotherapy appointment on October 30. The pain was still very much present from the surgery I had a mere six days ago, but thankfully, I still had the port. It was going to make this process so much easier, and I really needed easy now. So just like putting the nozzle of a gas hose into the opening of your car's gas tank, the nurse put the "hose" for the chemo into my port.

I thought, *I can do this. It's my last chemotherapy treatment! I won't have to do this ever again!*

My happiness and excitement seemed more powerful than the drugs. But of course, that night, the onslaught began when the drugs reared their ugly heads of power. Between the surgery's post-op pain that seared across my chest and the chemo's onslaught of stomach pain, nausea, and repeated sick episodes in the bathroom, I wasn't sure I was going to survive.

The next day, Bob drove me to get my IV for dehydration and nausea shot. They caused me to feel better and less nauseous, but the absence of the chemo side effects brought more attention to my healing chest.

Sadly, I had no immune system, but I sure did have lots of pain. It was undoubtedly a fight, but Bob was right beside me pulling me through. He refused to leave my side day or night.

He would try to bring some humor and make me laugh whenever he could by reminding me of some funny things we had done throughout our lives together.

"Remember the time when you were learning how to snow ski in Colorado, Evie?" he asked. "I was skiing with you because you were new to it. Then we went to get onto the chairlift, and I helped you sit down on it. It was transporting us up the hill, and as we got close to the top, you said, 'Okay, when it stops, help me off.' And I said, 'Honey, they don't stop. We have to ski off.'

I'll never forget the look you gave me. You started yelling, 'No, no, no! We can't ski off!' So I put my poles across you and said, 'Hold onto my ski pole.' I pulled you off, and we managed to ski off it together."

We both laughed and laughed at that memory and how I really thought those chairlifts would stop.

He would also tell me about funny things that happened to him on his trips or funny stories he had heard from someone else . . . anything to entertain me and make me laugh so that I could get my mind off my situation.

Still, I knew it was very difficult for him to see me go through all that. He, of all people, understood what I was feeling and thinking. As a result, he had the most compassion and credibility when it came to advice.

During those times, he would remind me, "Evie, honey, I survived this; you can survive it too. We've got this. We've got this together. We've got this with God. We've got this with friends. We've got this with family. You know we can do this. We've been here before, you and me, and we're still there together with my doctor appointments, and we're here with you with your appointments and recovery, and we'll be here with you for as long as you need."

Oh, how I appreciated his much-needed words of encouragement!

−45−

Just When You Think It's Over...

Just as I was gathering some strength from the beat-down of the surgery followed closely by my sixth chemo treatment, it was time to meet my radiologist, Dr. Sabrina Moore. When she walked into the exam room, the first thing that caught my eye was her dark curly hair as well as how young she appeared, yet she clearly knew what she was talking about. She answered every question and then some. I felt extremely confident with her.

"We have you scheduled for thirty-two radiation treatments," she announced. "Each one will last about half an hour."

I already knew what to expect with the radiation from all the treatments Bob had endured. Knowing too much can sometimes be a hazard, and for me right at that moment, it created fear. I saw what it had done to Bob, and he was much stronger than me.

"When do I start?" I asked timidly, not sure if I wanted her to answer.

Dr. Moore looked at her chart and said, "Your chest needs to heal more before we can begin. So we have you scheduled to preplan your radiation treatment on January 22, and the treatments will start on February 10."

I did some math in my head as to when I would be starting—in a little over two and a half months. I would be well over chemo, and hopefully, my chest would be healed as well. At least I wouldn't be going through chemo and radiation at the same time like Bob did. At least that was my thought and plan, but it didn't work out that way.

About two weeks after my last chemo treatment, I went to see Dr. Carson for an appointment.

She searched my face for a moment before saying, "Evelyn, I want you to go through three more chemotherapy treatments."

Shocked as a wave of nausea started developing, I managed to blurt out "What?"

Now it was my turn to search her face. I looked for any sign that she was playing a joke on me and a cruel one at that. There was no smile, no mischievousness in her eyes, only a professional demeanor with a fixed jaw that conveyed she stood firm in what she said.

"Why?" I asked, my tone argumentative and admittedly, miffed. "Why do I need more chemo? For heaven's sake, haven't I had enough?" Could she not see how burned out I was at this point?

"Evelyn, we need to make sure we got it all. Remember, we're fighting stage 3 triple-negative breast cancer. It's so aggressive, there's a strong chance it'll come back during the first five years after you're cancer free or in remission. However, if we do three more treatments, we can lessen that likelihood exponentially."

"I can't give you an answer now. I've got to go home and think about it and talk with Bob about it," I managed to respond.

I was so disappointed, actually, more like devastated! It was hard enough enduring the six hellish treatments, but now they wanted me to go through it three more times? In no way did I want that nor did I agree with it. The emotional and physical toll it had taken on my body was so much that I just didn't think I could take it anymore.

Bob and I talked back and forth about it. "I just can't, Bob. I just can't," I would cry. "Each and every time, I get so sick. I thought it was over. I went through the six treatments like a good little girl. I had my breasts cut off. But this? Well, this is overkill. I simply can't go through another round of their poison."

"I understand," Bob agreed. "I'm not sure that if they suggested I go through more radiation, I could do it either. But I want you to live, and I know you want to live. It's a tough decision to make. Why don't you talk with Jim Davis; see what he suggests."

Great idea! Dr. Jim Davis, our neighbor and friend and Bob's oncologist, had so much credibility with me. I would surely listen to his wisdom. Bob invited him over, and we presented my dilemma.

Bob asked, "Jim, if this was your wife, would you want her to go through three more treatments, to put even more poison into her body?"

"Yes, Bob, I would," he responded immediately and matter-of-factly.

I wasn't ready to throw in the towel just yet. "But I'm worried about all the poison being pumped into my body, that I'll never be able to detox from it," I argued, although there was a lot more to my aversion than detoxification.

His eyes softened. "Evie, I know my encouraging you to take three more treatments is not what you want to hear, but it's best." He studied my face as I tried to process his proclamation. "You can always detox your body after you're done with all this, but in the meantime, you need to take these additional treatments."

I needed that second opinion from a trusted professional. His confident response gave us the assurance to move forward, although unenthusiastically.

So the next day, I called Dr. Carson's office. "Schedule me for my next three chemo treatments."

And while I dreaded more chemo, things were moving so fast that I did have some victories. Two weeks after my surgery, I went to Dr. Stevens's office for her to remove my drains.

She said, "Okay, Evelyn, take a deep breath."

I complied, and she pulled them out. It only took a moment, and then they were out, gone!

Next, she removed my bandages. I had not seen my chest since before the surgery. I didn't know what I was expecting, but I surely didn't expect what I saw.

Lots of loose hanging skin had been left behind. Even though I knew my nipples would be removed and had tried to imagine what my chest would look like without them, I was surprised, and not in a good way.

It was all just too much to take in. I bawled right there in the doctor's office as Bob held me in his arms.

He said, "It's okay, honey. It doesn't look that bad."

I lifted my head off him and turned to the doctor. "Why is all this skin here? I mean, I knew there would be leftover skin, but I didn't expect this much. Why did so much get left behind?"

Her eyes softened. "We need all that extra skin to rebuild your new breasts, Evelyn, for when you have reconstructive surgery."

Oh yes! That made sense! Whew! They had told me about the excess skin, but I just had no idea the amount.

I forced myself to look at my chest again and studied them to find the positive. *Okay, I can adjust to no nipples. Once I have the reconstruction surgery, that excess skin will be put to good use.*

I came to the realization that it was all okay, no, it was more than okay; it was actually good that they were gone. Those beautiful breasts had a lethal invader that had tried to kill me, and now they and that murdering tumor were gone. They no longer had a chance to kill me. I had finally made peace with my breastless chest.

In that moment, gratitude overwhelmed me. I was alive, and that was most important. I vowed to serve God and to love my family with everything I had and that was within me. It would never be enough to thank my Savior for even being given a second chance at life, but for now, it was a start!

–46–

Miss Camo and Pearls

Time to let loose and live life. After all, that was what I was fighting for, and that was the opportunity my friend Sabrena Reed and her husband Brad were presenting to me.

Every year, they put on a fundraising event to support a charity. That year's affair was scheduled for November 15 and was called "Camo and Pearls."

Sabrena had called me at the beginning of October and announced, "We want you, Bob, and your dad to come. All the proceeds will be going to cancer research. You can sit at the front table with us. It'll be fun, Evelyn! Everyone has to dress up in camo or pearls. There will be a wonderful dinner and auction."

Of course, she had me at "cancer research." However, her invitation had been given prior to my surgery, so I couldn't give her a definitive yes, just a "let me see how I feel at that time" answer.

But when the time for the event came, Bob wanted to go and take me with him. "It's a great cause, one that we should support with everything we've gone through and are still going through," he stated.

I shook my head. "Sounds fun, but I'd rather not go this year. It's only been three weeks since my surgery, Bob, so I don't want to go looking horrible and deformed."

He gently took my hands in his, and in a loving tone, said, "Evie, it'll be good for you to get out among your friends."

He was right; we needed to support it, and I needed to get out. I took in a big breath and exhaled. "Okay, I'll go."

The night of the event, Bob wore jeans with a camo-print jacket that my dad had lent him. I wore jeans and Bob's old hunting vest that his dad had given him when he was a teenager. He had outgrown it as his muscles developed through the years from sports activities. The vest was kind of cool and even had a pocket for ammunition, but Bob never used it for that. He wasn't a hunter.

I didn't bother donning a wig. It was for cancer research, and my baldness was the result of treating my cancer. So I bared my skull with pride and accessorized it with a pair of pearl earrings and a camouflage scarf. I polished off my attire with a pearl necklace.

Bob eyes twinkled with approval as he looked me over. "You look so cute, Evie."

That perked me up and gave me the confidence I needed to get out in public and go somewhere other than a hospital, clinic, or doctor's office. We went to the event hoping for the best.

While sitting at our table, Sabrena stood up and looked at Bob. "Do you mind if I borrow your wife for a few minutes? I'll bring her back to you."

Bob nodded, and Sabrena took my hand.

"Follow me," she said.

Not knowing what Sabrena wanted, I shrugged and went along with whatever she had in mind. Next thing I knew, I was placed in the midst of other women who had formed a line leading up to a stage.

"What's this?" I asked Sabrena in utter confusion.

She raised her eyebrows and smiled. "Wait and see," she answered. "It's okay."

"But I'd rather sit down," I contended.

I turned to walk back to our table, but she grabbed

my hand to pull me back to her. "No, no. You gotta stay here."

A lady spoke into the microphone, which momentarily distracted me. "I want to welcome everyone here and thank all the ladies participating in our very first annual Miss Camo and Pearls Beauty Pageant."

I turned to look at Sabrena. "What?" I asked while trying to pull my hand away from hers.

But she held on tightly. "This will be good for you, Evelyn."

Not knowing what to do, I glanced over at our table and saw Bob, my dad, and Brad with big grins.

"I believe I've been set up," I stated, resigned to the fact that I was in that beauty pageant, like it or not.

The emcee asked each lady in line, one after the other, a question in front of the room that had hundreds of people.

I leaned over to Sabrena. "What am I supposed to do here?"

"The same thing they're doing. Just answer the question you're asked."

Ha! Easier said than done. I was super nervous

until I overheard two young girls talking to each other behind me.

One of them said, "I've never been in a beauty pageant. What am I supposed to do?"

The other girl replied, "Just smile and stick your chest out. It'll be okay."

Sabrena and I looked down at my chest and started laughing. It was the first real laugh I've had in a long time.

Then it was my turn. The emcee asked me, "If you had extra time, what would be your favorite thing to do?"

That was a no-brainer. I was a nature photographer, and I loved being outside. Without any hesitation, I felt confident with my answer. "I would be outside, photographing nature so that people can bring the beauty of nature into their homes."

I got a standing ovation and was consequently overwhelmed with humbleness and appreciation. Their reaction showed me that they didn't see me as a baldheaded, flat-chested cancer victim but as a strong person who loved the outdoors and nature.

While waiting for the judges to make their decision,

Sabrena and I stood on the stage, she holding my hand. I didn't know if her tight grip was to support me or to keep me in place so that I couldn't walk off the stage.

My cheeks started getting red from the discomfort of believing I shouldn't even be a participant in this pageant. There were so many beautiful women standing on that stage. I just wanted to leave and go back to my table.

Then the moment arrived for announcing Miss Camo and Pearls. The emcee started by saying, "Because of her strength, because of her beauty, and because of her love for nature, Miss Camo and Pearls 2013 is Evelyn Kormondy."

Everyone stood again and applauded as I made my way to the emcee to accept my winning sash. The embarrassment increased because I felt I had won because I had cancer.

As they put the crown and sash on me, I looked over at Bob. He was crying, clapping enthusiastically, and wearing the happiest smile ever! My dad and friends clapped and clapped as well.

After going back to my seat, Bob kissed me and declared, "I'm so proud of you. You did great! You looked so good and answered the question so well. You were overwhelmingly the winner."

Of course, Bob was a bit prejudiced.

Later on, I spoke to the judges, and they denied choosing me because of my condition. They said they did so because of my love for life and the outdoors.

I then had peace that I won fair and square. Before the contest, I had low self-esteem, believing I was now the ugly duckling. Sure, my friends and family thought I was beautiful, but reality told me differently because of what the treatments had done to me. But after that victory, I felt beautiful for the rest of the night.

It ended up being a wonderful evening with friends and one of Bob's and my best date nights during this recuperation time. It's hard to put into words the healing that comes after experiencing such normalcy in a time of turmoil.

When we got home, I was so exhausted. I think I stayed in bed for two days. Regardless, I was still Miss Camo and Pearls and will always be proud of that title.

– 4 7 –

The Last Chemo Treatment

Oh, how I dreaded this . . . another chemo treatment, especially when I thought about how it was supposed to be over. This was treatment number seven, and I still had two more to go after it. Was it even worth keeping count anymore?

This time around, however, Bob would be with me. Knowing that gave me comfort, but knowing what would happen a few hours later almost paralyzed me with fear. At least the worst would be over by next week when Thanksgiving arrived.

On the way to Mercy on that November 20 morning, I sat in the passenger seat preparing myself mentally and physically while Bob drove. I recalled how excited I was just three weeks ago to have chemo over and that part of Mercy in our rearview mirror. Now, it was in front of us . . . again.

That night didn't deviate from its pattern and

turned out to be another challenge. But thankfully, I felt better the next day, especially after my IV and nausea shot.

Then the time leading up to Thanksgiving was a blur and not too memorable. We went to my parents' house for dinner because I didn't feel too festive. But I wanted to recognize the holiday for what it was—Thanksgiving—and spend some precious time with my mom and dad.

Once Thanksgiving was over, we dove into the Christmas season. The house needed to be decorated, but I wasn't up to it. So Bob had some friends over, and together, they decorated the house and the tree.

I sat on the couch and stared at the ornaments hanging from it, remembering the story of my life etched upon each one. Sharing my stories with the girls while they were growing up, thus creating more layers of memories on top of them, was one of my favorite things about putting up the Christmas tree.

That year, though, I took it easy. I really didn't have much of a choice when on December 16, I underwent chemotherapy treatment number eight. I was an ole pro by now, bracing myself for the punch and kick to the stomach afterward. So that night, I planted myself on the bathroom floor until I was certain the toxins had finished ravaging my body. Bob was right there with me.

But then on December 22, he had to get back to work. He was working the Jacksonville Jaguars football game, so he didn't have to travel out of town. That was a huge blessing!

And I was able to watch the game from our loveseat and cheer our hometown team on!

As we lay in bed that night, he told me about some of the events that occurred at the game, making me feel as if I was there with him. I closed my eyes and envisioned everything he told me, every single detail. Then I thanked God for allowing us to spend another Christmas together.

On Christmas morning, the whole core family came to our house for our traditional Christmas breakfast of sliced ham and biscuits, hot cocoa, and coffee. Except for the biscuits our daughters prepared, my dad cooked everything else at his house and brought it all over. One reason was because of his wonderful chef abilities. The second was that the smells of most foods cooking made me nauseous.

Bob and I sat on our loveseat and watched the flurry of activities of everyone we were blessed to have in our home. Previously, we were always in the thick of it all. But for this year, Bob's and my part seemed to be relaxing while the others spoiled us.

Christmas turned out to be just wonderful with us all being together. We knew that love was most important that year, and it brought out my appreciation for being alive. *I was alive!* I just don't really think I can say that enough!

I embraced the privilege to be alive with such gratitude for our Savior's birth. He had been willing to come to this earth in human form to die on the cross so that we could have eternal life.

By the end of the day, I was completely worn out. It was all I could do to get out of bed the next day, but I forced myself to do so. Tomorrow, Bob would be leaving with two of our daughters to board a plane to Kapalua, Hawaii. He had to work the Hyundai Tournament of Champions scheduled for January 3–6, and he had accumulated enough frequent flyer miles to take the three girls and myself a week early for a mini family vacation. However, Michelle couldn't go because she had to work, but we had high hopes I could make it. Bob waited to buy my ticket until we knew for sure even though we both figured my chances of going were slim.

As it turned out, I was not medically approved to go. Regardless, I encouraged him to go with his other two girls, Kristy and Charlene. I didn't want them to miss out on the opportunity of spending some much-needed, much-deserved time with their dad after all that he had gone through.

While they were there, they sent me pictures. I studied each one with a smile on my face, longing to be there but knowing that we would go again someday.

We weren't able to spend New Year's Eve together either, so we tried to make the best of our separation by staying on the phone when the clock struck midnight on the East Coast even though Hawaii was five hours behind us. Bob lived in this time zone, and accordingly, 2014 had begun for him based on Eastern Standard Time.

When he returned on January 7, it was just in time for chemotherapy treatment number nine on January 8, my last and final one, well, so I had been told me. I just didn't know if I should believe them and if I should hope. I couldn't take another disappointment.

So Bob drove me there, stayed with me, and told me stories about his trip to Hawaii and made me laugh. The time went by fairly quickly as it always did with him there.

My sister Patty also came to this last treatment. She took a picture with all the kind nurses who had been involved with my treatments every time. We all shared in the joy of that final one and wore big smiles on our faces.

Carmen, the nurse who gave me most of my chemo, gave me a big hug and proclaimed, "I would love to see you again, sweetheart, but not for this. You come by and visit me anytime.

Bob and I drove home afterward light-hearted. I felt absolutely liberated! The festive atmosphere followed us into our home. We danced in the kitchen and celebrated this monumental milestone together.

And surprisingly, I didn't get sick that night like I had after previous treatments. Perhaps hope had evolved into reality, and that night, not even post-chemo nausea had a footing in my life!

–48–

My First Radiation Treatment

Time flies when you're having fun, well, for the most part. For the past three weeks, I had no treatments and only a few doctor appointments sprinkled in here and there.

Now it was time to get back down to the business of killing whatever cancer survived the poison of nine chemotherapy treatments and escaped the knife of surgery. Those cells had been evasive thus far, but my medical team was optimistic that radiation could eradicate the rest.

So on January 22, 2014, Bob and I met with my radiation oncologist, Dr. Moore, to map and preplan my treatment. Using pictures from my MRI, Dr. Moore showed me what could be described as a lighted grid and the areas they had targeted to radiate.

A nurse led me to another room so that I could be measured for a customized body mask to wear over my middle torso. Just like the mask Bob wore, both devices were intended to immobilize you during the treatment since the radiation beams needed to be precise in the locations they hit.

Afterwards, the nurse showed me a tube that looked like a snorkel. "This will help us help you with your breathing during radiation. You'll put this into your mouth. We'll tell you to take a deep breath and hold it. Then we'll let you know when you can breathe out."

I nodded and thought. *Simply don't breathe, Evelyn. Don't breathe when they're giving you radiation.*

Not breathing for periods of time seemed to be important. Because it's not something I normally do, I made a mental note that before radiation began, I needed to practice holding my breath and timing it for as long as I could.

At the end of the appointment, I met with Dr. Moore again. She wanted to make sure I didn't have any more questions.

"Thirty-two treatments, right?" I clarified.

She nodded. "Yes, thirty-two. As you know, the first one's on Monday, February 10 at 9:00 in the morning."

"Right. February 10," I confirmed in a tone reflecting my dread even though we all knew it was necessary. "It's on my calendar."

In fact, all thirty-two treatments were written down on my calendar. I wanted the satisfaction of marking each one off as I completed them.

The nurse handed me the final schedule. My eyes traveled to the last one—yep, Wednesday, March 26. That coincided with my calendar. Whether it was my treatments or Bob's, seeing that last day always gave me hope, something to look forward to.

But in the meantime, I had to endure thirty-two treatments. Although I was in a hurry to mark them off my calendar, February 10 came much too soon. I was back at Mercy before I knew it.

It seemed like yesterday that I had been plagued with chemotherapy, and now, radiation therapy was going to have its way with me. This was part of the process I had been dreading the most after seeing firsthand how it affected Bob.

Not long after getting checked in, I was called back and led to the area where I was to change out of my clothes and into one of their gowns. So many questions, thoughts, and emotions swirled through my mind and then turned into an ominous feeling that weighed heavily on me as I wrapped the gown around me. Would my treatments be as severe as Bob's or less? It made sense that the burn wouldn't be as bad since he had radiation twice a day, and I would only have it once.

Remember, you're not going to feel the hurt for several treatments, I reminded myself. *It's going to be painless.*

I focused hard on tying the gown closed while continuing to ponder the situation in front of me. Then as soon as I stepped out of the dressing room, fear overwhelmed my reassuring self-talk, and sheer nervousness made me sick to my stomach.

Hesitantly, I walked into the hallway and spotted Bob standing next to a closed door. The anxiety built with each step.

As I approached him, he raised his eyebrows and asked, "Ready?"

Was anyone ever ready to be shot with radiation? I nodded anyway.

Bob opened the door and led me into the therapy room. By now, he knew the layout by heart. He stood to the side as the staff got me prepared, just like I had done two years earlier when he was the one on the table.

The radiation oncology technician ladies were so kind and sensitive to my needs. They didn't want me to feel more exposed than necessary, so they didn't lower my gown until they had to leave the room. When they did, Bob followed them.

Panic set in. The technician started talking to me on the intercom to calm me down and piped in '70s music overhead. It helped me to relax, knowing I wasn't alone.

Then he played "Day by Day," and I sang along in my head. It put my focus on God and centered me.

Next came the radiation. I took in a deep breath each time they commanded. Then they would say, "Hold it . . . hold it . . . hold it."

I did, but my chest burned and felt as if it was about to burst. Still, I couldn't give in to the compulsion to let it out no matter what. The radiation had to have the maximum amount of positive impact and the least amount of negative side effects.

I must hold it . . . I must! I kept telling myself.

It seemed as if I had to hold it for minutes, but in reality, it was more like seconds. Regardless, each and every one of those seconds was terrifying. To dispel the fear, I would imagine myself lying there peacefully and praying to God.

And finally, it was over. Actually, once I calmed down, time went by rather quickly. As I was leaving the therapy room, I glanced at the clock . . . about thirty minutes total including prep time.

I was so happy to be changing into my clothes, but mostly, I was relieved. One radiation treatment down; thirty-one to go. And it wasn't as bad as I had made it in my mind. Tomorrow, I would be back, but I would be okay. The fear of the unknown had left the building.

Bob greeted me in the waiting room. He was so happy to see me, and I was so glad he was with me for this first time.

On the drive home, he asked, "How did it go?"

I glanced down at my hands in my lap and then back up and through the front window. "The hardest part was holding my breath for so long, but the music and staff made it easier." I tried to keep my response light.

Bob looked at me briefly and then he put his eyes back on the road. "When I was out in the waiting room, I thought about what you were going through. It was difficult knowing you were getting the same kind of treatments I did." He took in a deep breath and then exhaled. "I know what they're like."

We came to a red light and stopped. Although I was staring straight ahead, pondering the cumulative effect that was to come, I could see him out of the corner of my eye watching me.

I couldn't say much. We both knew that it would be a controlled burn, that these treatments were smooth at first, but then they would get worse. As my protector, he didn't want me to go through what he did. If he could, he would go in there and take those treatments for me so that he could shield me from them.

But we also knew he couldn't do that. The cancer had attacked *me* this time around, not him, and ultimately, it was my battle to fight.

Instead, he had to settle for encouraging me and taking care of my wounds that would surely come. He decided to stay in town to see me through my first week of radiation. Plus, Valentine's Day was on Friday, and he wanted to spend it with me.

"What do you want to do for Valentine's Day?" he asked.

When that day came, although I had only undergone four treatments, I didn't feel like going out to dinner, didn't look like I should go out to dinner, and didn't feel like eating anything.

"Why don't we watch Valentine movies on Hallmark?" I suggested.

He agreed. That night, Bob fixed me a bowl of applesauce (my favorite at that time) with a bow wrapped around it. Over dinner, he talked more about all the places we had travelled and the places we still wanted to go together. He made me laugh, and he reminded me of our dreams, of the things we still wanted to do.

Afterwards, he turned on the TV and switched over to the Hallmark Channel. We sat down on our loveseat and held hands. I was happy, satisfied, and content.

As the movie began to play, I was reminded that it's those little things in life that are the best things that you can do for each other. It's knowing that each other is there, and at the end of the day, that's all we really ever need.

−49−

The Slow Burn

My mother had a stroke the next day. It wasn't the first one either. After each of them, however, she had always sprung back with minor damage. It was easier—preferable—to believe that this time would be no different.

But this time, it was.

I visited her during those first two days, that Saturday and Sunday, and it was difficult to watch her decline. She had always been so strong, raising six daughters, being a grandmother to six granddaughters and a great-grandmother to great-granddaughters and a great-grandson. Through it all, her beauty never waned nor did her remarkableness.

Then I had to get back to my own battle on Monday. With four treatments under my belt thus far, I refused to let these radiation treatments consume my life. Sure, I had to move things around to make the appointments as most people would do for any appointment, but I still nevertheless went through with my daily activities.

Upon arriving at Mercy, I would suit up, which for me meant donning a hospital gown, and head for the treatment room to be shot with radiation time and again.

I would lie on the table and sing along in my head to the '70s tunes that resonated from the speakers or to my song "Day by Day." My mind would wonder to Bob in the waiting room if he was in town, and if not, to him shooting whatever golf tournament or sporting event at the time. It was hard on him. I could only imagine what was going through his mind when he envisioned what I was going through.

Next, I would think about our daughters and my family and how I would do anything to survive so that I could have more time with them here on this earth.

Then before I knew it, the tech would announce over the intercom that they were done. It became routine, something I did with my eyes shut.

The treatments were more of a nuisance than anything else. I still didn't feel any sensation—good, bad, or indifferent—during it and after it, and I had yet to experience any side effects. I went home and on with my life, not thinking anymore about radiation until I would have to return the next day for another treatment.

But radiation therapy, it's sneaky. It's like the story of the proverbial frog—If you put a frog in boiling water, it will jump out. But if you put the frog in a pot of tepid water and slowly turn up the heat, it will boil to death.

I was the latter frog. I had been put in a pot of tepid water—no big deal—and the cumulative effect of the radiation was gradually turning up the heat. I wasn't going to boil to death, but after a while, I would feel like I was.

We all knew it was a matter of time.

But I was tough. Maybe, just maybe, I would escape its full wrath. But after about the tenth treatment, my neck and chest started turning red as if I had gotten sunburned from being at the beach for too long.

Subsequently, I started noticing the shortness of breath and the accompanying fatigue. It didn't come as a surprise because of my on-the-job training with Bob's radiation. It had been a great teacher but the kind you really hated. She started off nice and sweet, but as the school year continued, she reared her ugly head, and oh, could she be viscous!

What I had learned from our history with radiation was what no one could see—the damage occurring beneath the surface. Sure, the radiation was killing the cancer, but it was also damaging other parts of my body, including my lungs and heart.

Then after each treatment, I would go to my parents' home to check on my mother and to be with her. As I had already figured out, this last stroke ended up being much bigger than the previous ones. She became even more weak and had trouble walking.

At the end of February when we were with her, she looked up at me from her bed and smiled. "Evie," she started, "can you see the angels? Aren't they beautiful?"

Her questions were comforting while at the same time, they confirmed to me that she wasn't going to make it this time around.

Sadly, hospice had to be brought in that first week of March. They took care of her and kept us updated as to her condition. Then when it was close to the time of her passing, they let us know.

On Thursday, March 6, 2014, the family gathered around my precious mother as she lay in bed. Her eyes remained closed as she rested. We all knew it would be any moment, and extreme grief could be felt in the atmosphere. We held her hand, talked to her, and sang gospel music. I believe it comforted her; I know it comforted me.

As I stared at her, realizing she would be leaving me soon, I tried to focus on the fact that she would be going to heaven where she would no longer be in pain. Until then, we wanted her to know how much we honored her and who she was. The result was an unbelievable amount of love that spread throughout the room.

My dad knelt next to her bed. He held her hand and told her he loved her.

Surprisingly, after two days with her eyes closed, she opened them and smiled at my dad. "I love you," she whispered to him.

He moved his face close to hers and gave her a kiss. I couldn't help but smile through my tears as I was privileged to witness the depth and beauty of my parents' love for each other.

Then she took her last breath. It was surreal. This strong woman was gone. A deluge of tears now flooded my eyes. Thankfully, Bob had been standing behind me, and he wrapped his arms around me for support.

Going through that loss and seeing my father so brokenhearted overwhelmed me with sorrow. My mother had been his true love like Bob was my true love, so I could understand his pain to a certain degree; however, I couldn't imagine my life without my Bob.

I prayed for God to watch over Daddy. I loved him so much and knew Mom and my sister Scottie Bryan were in heaven watching over him and me. But as children of God, Dad and I had within us that blessed assurance that one day, we would see them again in heaven where we would all be united! That kind of peace is priceless . . . and healing!

For radiation, well, it never stopped for anything, not even to grieve the death of a parent. The next day, Friday, I was back at the hospital at 8 a.m. sharp for another round.

By 8:30, I scurried out the door and headed to my parents' house to help with the preparations. Fortunately, my treatments were early enough in the morning that I was able to attend her service later in the afternoon.

Afterward, I was left alone to deal with my own grief. It was a journey I would walk with bittersweet tears. The bitter part came from knowing I would always miss my mother . . . always! She had left a void in my heart that would never be filled. The sweet part came from knowing she was in a better place, made complete and whole, no more pain, and she was now dancing with Jesus on streets of gold!

Everything was going to be okay, but it would be a process to get to that point. Emotionally, I would heal from my loss of Mom. Physically, my body would heal as well. Despite everything, my strength would be returning, and soon, I would remember how good it felt to take a deep breath again.

All in due time . . .

But spiritually, I had grown and was so much stronger. All was well with my soul.

–50–

The Final Time

March 26, 2014—my thirty-second and final radiation treatment!

This last one wasn't only about completing all of the necessary cancer treatments I had to endure over the previous nine months. It was about reaching a hugely significant milestone that gave me permission to move on with my life.

Sure, there would be follow-up doctor appointments and routine tests and imaging to see if my lungs remained clear. And my next hurdle was the reconstruction surgery. But at that point, although I dreaded another surgery, I considered it to be one of many steps to reclaiming my life and preparing for my future.

Oh yes, I had a future!

So that morning, I had a pep in my step as I held Bob's hand on the walkway leading to that radiation clinic for the last time. It didn't matter that I was in pain from the sensation of having a really bad sunburn that worsened with each day; it was the last treatment. Period! The boxes on the checklist had been almost all checked off, and the feeling of satisfaction for completing such a feat was euphoric. More important was my deep and profound appreciation to my Savior for keeping me through it all.

During that final time of lying on that table, I held my breath upon command. They still reminded me not to move, but I did it all with a smile. I sang "Day by Day" in my head louder than I ever had and proclaimed, "Day by day, oh dear Lord, we made it through!"

When I walked back into the waiting room that last time, Bob stood up from his chair with a big smile on his face. He started applauding me for making it through. It was a beautiful moment.

The icing on the cake, though, was walking up to the bell and the giddiness that emerged from the realization that it was finally my turn to ring it.

However, the sweet taste of victory was dampened during the following two weeks after completing radiation. That's when the real burning started. The "sunburn" sensation evolved into a super-bad sunburn. About five days post-radiation, it felt like I had third-degree burns across my neck, chest, and left arm. The skin actually peeled off.

It hurt so much that lotion would need to be applied frequently. I couldn't do it by myself because it was under my arm, around my back, and up my neck on the left side. The removal of those lymph nodes made it impossible to reach those areas.

When Bob was out of town, my dear friend Kathy came over twice a day to put the lotion on those badly burned wounds. Although she was gentle, I would still cry from her touching those raw areas. It was always a bit embarrassing to expose myself to someone else both emotionally with my pain and physically with my wounds.

Fortunately with Kathy, she would reassure me and say, "Don't be embarrassed, Evelyn. It's okay; I'm your friend."

And when she couldn't come, my daddy did.

The intense pain kept me from sleeping at night. If I put myself in a certain position, I would at least nod off, but then the pain would wake me back up. I became so exhausted from not sleeping as well as dealing with the agony on a constant basis that functioning became more than challenging.

While walking to the shower one day, I stopped and stared at myself in the mirror. No breasts. No hair. Burns across my neck and what was left of my now-flat chest. Depends underwear.

Who are you? I asked my reflection. *I don't recognize you, and I no longer know you.*

This is what cancer does—it steals its victim's identity and turns them into someone or something else they do not recognize.

Then I reminded myself, *Evie, this is only temporary. Cancer's time in your body had its run, but thanks to God and your medical team, it was short-lived.*

This fight had ultimately gone beyond the physical realm that involved chemotherapy, surgery, and radiation. It had barged smack-dab into the spiritual realm where my weapons of warfare were many—praying, reading His Word, and as long as I had breath, praising Him. I utilized all my weapons to the fullest extent. As a result, the plan to take me down backfired big time! I knew that by the grace of God, I would come through it. He had held me so far, and He always finishes what He starts.

Then as quickly as the burns intensified, they were healed. That was a true gift from God.

Altogether, the burning pain probably lasted a couple of weeks, but again, it was worth it. I would never have to suffer through the effects of radiation again.

Afterwards and over the course of the next several months, I began pulling my life back together to resume my pre-cancer norm. It was a slow process, but I was blessed to have that process at whatever speed it was given.

I had gotten used to my bald head. My wigs were beautiful, but I still wanted my own hair. Every morning, I would check my scalp for any sign of new growth. When my scalp stopped feeling smooth and some peach fuzz started appearing, I got so excited because I realized my follicles were alive and well and pushing forth hair!

Another activity I was eager to return to was travelling with Bob. Maybe by the time I was physically able, I would have hair.

But I still grieved the loss of my breasts, so my doctors referred me to Dr. Tina Maxwell, a psychologist, to help me cope. I ended up seeing her three or four times, and it helped. She was an understanding and wise person to talk with outside of my family.

Dr. Carson continued seeing me every two weeks to see how everything was going for me and if I was experiencing any side effects. I was—neuropathy in my feet. They would tingle and burn as pain would shoot through them. Sometimes, it was impossible to walk on them because they hurt so bad. I learned that I could no longer walk barefoot, and that if I walked on my feet all day, the pain worsened at night.

But I looked at the big picture and therefore, refused to let that distract me from my joy of living! It was just another life adjustment from surviving cancer!

To my surprise, I also developed lymphedema, a swelling in the arm or leg or in both arms or legs due to a blockage in the lymphatic system or an inability for the fluid to escape from the body. I started noticing it about eight months after my double mastectomy.

Even though the doctors had forewarned me about this possible side effect of the surgery, at this point, I really thought I was in the clear. In fact, I figured I wasn't going to have much more happen to me in terms of side effects for a lot of things. And I certainly didn't think a whole lot about lymphedema. But it can creep up on a person without notice.

I didn't think anything about the swelling in my arm, so thank God for my sister Shirley! She came to visit me one day. As a trained and certified lymphedema specialist with a focus on its treatment, she immediately recognized this swelling for what it was—lymphedema.

Shirley took me to a local company so that they could measure me for a customized lymphedema sleeve to wear. It had to fit snugly from the hand all the way up the arm to both reduce the current swelling as well as prevent any future swelling. It was a device that I would need to wear for many years to come, especially if I wanted to travel with Bob. The change in air pressure while flying in a plane would make this sleeve a requirement.

While waiting for the company to create my sleeve, Shirley would treat the swelling on a regular basis with special lymphedema bandages that she wrapped around my fingers all the way up my arm when needed. Because of her love and care, I was truly blessed to keep my lymphedema at stage 1 with her help.

Then the local company called me to let me know my sleeve was finished. They asked me to come in and try it on. Shirley went with me to ensure it fit correctly.

While there, the technician mentioned that I might want to consider a prosthetic bra.

I didn't see that coming! A prosthesis is custom-created to replace a missing body part, and in my case, the missing body part, or parts, were my breasts. They wanted to create a prosthesis to replace my breasts until I could have reconstruction surgery.

After considering my options and realizing it would be another three months before I would have breasts, I went ahead and purchased one. My prosthetic bra was created, and I started wearing it, but I found it uncomfortable.

That was okay. I ditched the bra for several reasons. One was for comfort, and another was because I was who I was meant to be, which was why I wasn't always keen on wearing a wig to cover up my baldness. I would when the occasion merited it, but for the most part, I preferred to bare my shiny head to the world.

So if I felt that way about my bald head, imagine how I felt about my flat chest. To me, strap-on breasts were worse. Although I didn't bare them to the world, I knew they weren't real. They didn't feel natural to me because they weren't natural.

In just a few more months, I would get my own breasts anyway. I would be able to reclaim control over my life and appearance soon enough.

And when I did, I would be me again!

− 51 −

Reconstruction Surgery #1

I had made it to June 20, the one-year anniversary of my official "more-than-likely" diagnosis of cancer. A year ago seemed like a lifetime ago, and in a way, it was. The year before, I was a different Evelyn. Since then, I had been in the battle for my life against a formidable foe—an aggressive form of cancer.

As fast as I seemed to be running through this journey, there were a few events that seemed to be dragging on longer than I liked. The removal of my port was one of them.

By July 5, 2014, it had been in for over one year, long after my chemotherapy had ended. Every time I would ask to have it removed, Dr. Carson would say, "Let's keep it in in case you need to have more chemo."

I wasn't happy with her decision. I wanted this device out of my body. In my mind, when I'm done, I'm done!

It didn't matter what I wanted, though. At the time, that port wasn't going anywhere. So I might as well buckle myself in and hurry up and wait.

On the upside, my hair was growing back, although very slowly. Every once in a while, I would put on a scarf or wig while it crept its way out of my scalp.

I was told that when your hair comes back, it can be different than what it had been before chemo. It can be thinner, and the color can be different.

Well, I found out that was all true. My hair color changed drastically. It went from red to white with some gray, an interesting combination. Bob loved it, but I found the adjustment hard, so I continued to wear my red wig. I had lost so many of my physical attributes that I wanted some kind of semblance of me when I looked in the mirror.

By the time mid-July 2014 rolled around, I evidently must have accomplished retaining or reclaiming some kind of likeness to my former self. I was surprised when someone from my past recognized me, even though I was still fairly bald.

It happened while I was with Bob in Lake Tahoe for the annual celebrity golf tournament. I had finished all my treatments months ago and was feeling so much stronger. We had even asked Dr. Carson whether she thought I would be okay going to this event, and she did.

She was right. The plane ride was no problem and neither was the drive from the airport. The high altitude didn't seem to bother me at all. So far, so good. Consequently, I managed to walk down to the golf course and watch the tournament.

Then Charles Barkley walked by. I waved at him and said, "Hi, Mr. Barkley."

He stopped and studied me for a moment. At first, he didn't seem to remember who I was. The last time he saw me was when I had red hair and stood inside the lines as a photographer. Now I stood with the other spectators, and my red hair was covered with a scarf.

Then his eyes showed recognition as a grin spread across his face. "Little Voice?" he asked.

I returned his grin and nodded my head. "Yes, sir."

He strolled over to me. "Where have you been, Little Voice? What happened?"

"Well, I got diagnosed with cancer about thirteen months ago." My fingers involuntarily touched the scarf on the sides of my head. "I'm sorry I missed you last year. I was here, but I couldn't walk down to the tournament." Then I continued to tell him more of my story.

He gave me one of his great big bear hugs and went on his way. Seeing him again, his recognition of me, the hug he gave me, his sincere interest in wanting to know how I was doing, it all made my day. What a kind man!

If Charles Barkley could figure out who I was, then I must be getting Evelyn back. There were still some other attributes I needed to recoup to finish the job, though, or at least get as close to them as possible.

Of course, I would never get my breasts back, but I would get the next best thing during my upcoming reconstruction surgery. The results would be different like my hair growth was, but unlike my new hair color, this difference was going to be determined by me; the changes would be my decision.

On September 02, a little over six weeks after Tahoe, Bob and I met with Dr. Paine, the plastic surgeon. Now that the reconstruction surgery, a life-changing event, was before us, it held our primary focus. We were on a fact-finding mission.

The last time we had met with this doctor eleven months ago, this surgery seemed so surreal at that time, so far away in the future. I was still having chemo, and my double mastectomy hadn't even taken place. Dr. Paine had introduced us to our choices for the first time, and we had made our decisions from *that* perspective.

Since then, I had many opportunities to talk with other women about their choices, some similar to mine, some different, as well as do some research to determine which would be best for my body type. Now, we wanted . . . *needed* to make sure that I had all available options in front of me. Plus, the last time we had met, my brain fog kept me from fully understanding everything. My mind was much more lucid during this appointment, and things would make much more sense.

So Bob and I wanted to discuss all the options again and make sure we understood them clearly. Then we wanted to further discuss details about the upcoming surgery.

Dr. Paine's appearance to seemingly know a lot about breast reconstruction and what I wanted made me excited that I had decided to go through with it. He was going to be good; I just knew it. I also appreciated how he had given Bob and me choices during our first visit, ones that we could make instead of them being made for us. By this time, having a voice mattered.

When I arrived for my appointment, his waiting room was almost standing room only like it had been when we met almost a year ago.

Wow, I thought, *he still has a lot of patients. He must be really good because so many people obviously trust him. No wonder Dr. Stevens had highly recommended him; she knew how good he was from working with him lots of times.*

The wait didn't seem too bad—another plus for Dr. Paine. Then he came into my room, and he had quite the bedside manner. We reviewed the choices that Bob and I had made during our last visit.

He told us about the different kinds of procedures to rebuild the breasts. We asked questions, but it was a lot to ponder.

Bob cut through our confusion by asking, "What kind of procedure would you recommend for Evelyn, Dr. Paine?"

He glanced at me and then back at Bob. "The best procedure would be a latissimus dorsi flap on the left side where the cancer was," he suggested. Then his eyes shifted onto me. "What happens is that I'll take muscle from your upper back and turn it sideways, bring it under your arm, and rebuild your breast with that muscle and the saline implant. It's not an easy surgery, but I think it will work out well. On the right side, we'll insert an implant under the muscle."

I nodded, already feeling the pain. Regardless, I agreed that his recommendation was the best procedure for me. The way he explained it made sense. He would use the muscle from my back, turn it, and bring it around to the front. The muscle would still be connected to my back.

If I was going to endure all that, though, I wanted to make sure he remembered what we had discussed (and debated) eleven months ago—my new cup size. It was important enough to repeat my desire to make sure he understood nothing had changed—*I did not want a D-cup size. Please make me a small C-cup!*

So I said, "As a reminder, Dr. Paine, when you reconstruct my breasts, I want a small C-cup size like we decided upon the last time I was here."

He jotted down some notes. I presumed they included my cup-size preferences.

Then he gave a nod and said, "We need to make an appointment with you beforehand to insert the tissue expanders."

"What's involved with that?" I asked. "Will it hurt?"

He smiled and shook his head. "Nah. We do this procedure at Crestview Hospital. We put you in a twilight sleep and then place the expanders under the skin, which are actually empty breast implants. Then you'll come back to my office every week so that we can inject them with saline. You may think you have a lot of excess skin, but it's still not enough. These injections will gradually stretch your skin to your perfect cup size. These injections only take a moment."

I nodded again as I tried to process all this information. That night, I talked about my visit with Bob. We prayed, wanting to make sure we had made the right decisions.

The next morning, I called the scheduling nurse at Dr. Paine's office to inform her that we were ready to move forward with the reconstruction surgery and for her to give me a date for it.

"Okay, Mrs. Kormondy," she said, "we can get you in on October 24.

Oh wow!" I exclaimed. "On October 24, one year ago, I had my double mastectomy."

"That's so interesting!" the nurse exclaimed. "Between your mastectomy and your reconstruction surgery, I bet that's one date you'll never forget." She chuckled and paused for a moment. "Okay, now that we've settled upon the date of your surgery, let's go ahead and schedule your saline injections too."

I scribbled down the dates she had given me for the next six weeks. Afterward, I studied my calendar and sighed with happiness and contentment. I had a lot to look forward to after almost fifteen months of hell.

And the victories didn't only involve my reconstruction surgery. Dr. Stevens had announced (after much prodding and pleading) that she was removing my port. Woo-hoo! She didn't have to tell me twice.

Two days later on September 04, I couldn't get to her office fast enough.

When Dr. Stevens went to remove the port, however, she found that it had been in there for so long that adhesions had grown around it. As a result, removing it was more challenging and took more time than any of us had expected.

And it hurt. It wasn't like when they had put it in. Then, I was in a twilight sleep, but not for this procedure; I was wide awake! They only applied a numbing agent, which I assumed was sufficient if taken out before the adhesions. But with the adhesions, I surely felt it!

Once she finally removed that port, it was so worth it! It was now gone. Its void represented more than the removal of a plastic gadget; it represented that cancer was in my rearview mirror.

I now have a small scar on the upper right side of my chest that reminds me of power, survival, strength, and beauty. It's a scar I acquired during the fight for my life and how I came out the victor in this battle through Jesus Christ my Savior!

The next battle was the reconstruction surgery. Once that was over and done, I envisioned holding up my arms in both victory and praise.

The next week, I went to the hospital to have Dr. Paine insert my tissue expanders. After it was over, it didn't really hurt, just felt odd due to how tight that area now was.

But with each visit and injection, it did start to hurt. It felt like he kept adding more saline than necessary.

My skin got tighter and tighter, and the pain increased more and more as he expanded the skin.

Bob happened to be home for about three weeks during these saline injections, which allowed me to have a set of objective eyes. This was too close and personal with me, and I didn't want to make any decisions or observations of what may be my obsessive scrutiny of my own soon-to-be breasts. We are all our biggest critics, discovering things that most people don't notice. But I knew Bob would give me an honest and sincere evaluation.

"Bob," I started, "don't you think they're too big? He filled up these bags so much that they're stretching the skin too much."

He studied them and agreed. He then went with me to my next appointment, which happened to be the next day.

"Dr. Paine," Bob said, "this isn't the size Evelyn wants. We've discussed it, and she wants a small C-cup."

The doctor responded, "Mr. Kormondy, I have to make it larger because I need room to work with my design. I'm like an artist working with clay."

That made sense, and what did Bob and I really know about the matter? We trusted the doctor to know what he was doing. After all, he had come highly recommended.

−52−

They're Not Right!

For sure, I had endured a lot of stress over the past three years. It was naïve to think I would be able to continue dealing with it, which really meant pushing it deep down inside as I smiled at the world.

Consequently, over the previous week, I had been experiencing moments when my heart would race. I reported this to Dr. Stevens, and she made an appointment for me to see Dr. Benjamin Jones, a cardiologist. He ordered a heart monitor for me to wear for a twenty-four-hour period. So before I went into surgery, actually before anyone goes into a surgery, any heart problems should be made known.

On September 24, exactly one month before my reconstructive surgery, I went to pick up the heart monitor. The tech taped the leads onto my chest and gave me a satchel-like bag in which to carry the monitor.

I returned to the cardiac center the next day to return the monitor. Fortunately, no problems were noted. We all concluded that those moments when my heart raced were due to the anxiety that kept cropping up.

Thank you, Jesus!

Now I could move forward with my reconstruction surgery with peace!

And I did! On the morning of October 24, 2014, I woke up at home like I did other mornings. Then it hit me that my reconstruction surgery was that day. Fear overcame me because I wasn't sure about what I was getting myself into. Should I have left it alone and lived my life without breasts? What were they going to look like? Better than the ones I used to have? Worse?

Then excitement replaced fear at the thought of looking just like me again. Of course, they wouldn't look like my other breasts, but that was okay; those had tried to kill me. These new ones were going to be improved and in my desired size.

Once we arrived at the hospital, my emotions resorted back to being mixed—excitement about restoring my life and trepidation about enduring another surgery. All in all, the excitement won out because the outcome would enable me to take back a part of my identity that the cancer had robbed from me.

Bob held my hand before they wheeled me back. "You okay, Evie?" he asked in his loving tone.

I forced a smile and nodded. "I'm okay."

When the nurse came to give me something to relax me, I became very nervous. I didn't really want to go to sleep because I was afraid.

Bob prayed with me. Right then, I knew that God would be in the surgery with me, holding me and guiding the surgeon's hand.

So I took a deep breath and relaxed. That was all I remembered until I woke up in recovery. I was quickly reminded why I hated undergoing surgery. The grogginess from the anesthesia was initially miserable, but it was nothing compared to the pain.

Oh well, I had been down this road before. Fortunately, I could go home straight from the recovery room. No overnight stays and monitoring.

Then it was back to the drains for not only me, but also for Bob. This time, though, we knew what to expect.

As it was with Dr. Stevens, Dr. Paine scheduled several post-op visits where he would check the drains and replace the bandages. During those visits, I reported my pain to him. He would respond, "Well, there's going to be pain for a little while, Evelyn. Your body has to heal. It just went through major surgery."

I couldn't argue at this point. Pain was part of the process, a big consequence of surgery that I would have to deal with while I healed. I mean, I assumed I was healing.

Finally after a couple of weeks post-surgery, Dr. Paine removed the drains and bandages. And as with Dr. Stevens, oh, what a wonderful day that was!

But then I got to see my breasts for the first time. They were huge! My jaw dropped in shock.

"Dr. Paine," I said, turning to face him, "what happened? They're not right. They're much bigger than I had told you I wanted them to be."

He waved his hand toward me, dismissing my concern. "Oh, that's to be expected. They're swollen right now. Let the bruising and swelling come down, and they'll be fine."

I didn't know any different than to trust him. After

all, I had talked to him many, many times about what I wanted in terms of size, and he had always seemed to listen. Surely, they were just swollen. *Whew!* I simply needed to be patient.

And I was. I waited and waited for a couple more weeks, realizing I needed to give it time. But I would often look at my breasts in the mirror, and I wouldn't see any change in their size.

One night after staring at my reflection, I rushed out of the bathroom into our bedroom where Bob was sitting in bed reading a book. "Look, Bob." I showed him my breasts. "They're still not right. This wasn't what I expected. One of my breasts is a double D, and the other one is an double E." I started sobbing.

I could feel that the expanders had been placed too far into my chest, which increased the pain. In fact, on the left side where the cancer was, the expander was not only placed too far forward, but it also extended to the side under my arm, making me feel like a bulked-up bodybuilder who can't put their arm all the way down against their side. It was obvious that they were too big.

My next appointment with Dr. Paine was the next

day, which was November 20. I wanted to get this over with. Bob went with me so that we could talk to him together face to face.

"Dr. Paine, what happened here?" I asked, trying hard to keep my cool. "They are way too big. Plus, they're two different sizes!"

He assessed them for a few moments before responding. "Evelyn," he said, "they're not two different sizes. It's just the swelling. I do see a bit of unevenness, but I can go back in again and do another surgery. We'll get this right, and you'll be happy," he assured me.

I looked at Bob as so many questions ran through my brain. *We'll go in for another surgery? We'll get this right? Why didn't we get this right the first time? Why would you put me through this again? Why didn't you listen to me all those times when I told you what I wanted?*

I was so angry!

His office scheduled my next surgery for May 29, 2015. I would have to endure large and uneven breasts for another six months. Aggravating, but my body did need a break . . . and so did my anger.

– 5 3 –

Reconstruction Surgery #2

"I do *not* want such big implants, Dr. Paine." I insisted during my pre-op visit for reconstruction surgery number two. "It's very important to me to be a small C-cup please."

He nodded with a smile on his face just like he did the last time, yet here I was with the wrong size and by a lot. His confident expression made me believe he was listening and understood. However, when a woman says she wants a small C-cup yet a double D and a double E were instead given, someone wasn't listening, no matter how many times it was stated.

Dr. Paine proceeded to measure the size of my breasts so that during surgery, he could replace the implants that were too big with smaller ones and trim the skin so that everything would like nice, at least that was the plan, so I thought.

Then May 29 arrived, the long-awaited date to

correct the mistakes from my first reconstruction surgery. It wasn't soon enough for me. I wanted this debacle finally fixed.

By now, Bob and I were used to the routine: Whoever wasn't having surgery went into the kitchen and made themselves a cup of coffee. The one scheduled for surgery was prohibited from consuming anything, including liquids.

Next, we would pray. We would give each other a hug. The nonpatient would look at the patient and say, "Honey, you've got this. Go and get it done."

We would leave the house early, and Bob would drive regardless of who was having surgery. This time, surgery was scheduled for 7:30 that morning.

The drive to the hospital, which was closer to our house than Mercy, was quiet. I stared out the passenger door window and pondered my situation. Chemotherapy, double mastectomy, radiation treatments . . . I thought the most challenging fight against breast cancer was well behind me. However, my biggest fight turned out to be the reconstruction surgery. Who would have thought, but the size was over the top. Post-surgery cramps in my left breast and under my arm were way too prevalent.

I thought we would have been done with this whole experience at this point. Not so fast . . . Here I was, having Bob drive me to the hospital again for another surgery to fix the subpar work of this surgeon.

Shaking my head, I could feel the frustration rising up again. I couldn't believe I was having to go through this another time. And then more drains, more pain, and less time living a normal life.

What if he gets it wrong again? I was so tired of being poked and prodded. It was emotionally, mentally, and physically exhausting.

At this point, all I could do was put it in God's hands. So I prayed silently and asked God to guide the surgeon's hands, to remind him what I wanted done and what needed to be done.

In a few hours, it would all be over. Bob would drive me home and take care of me. I would be groggy from the anesthesia, so I would rest for the remainder of the day. Then the pain would re-emerge, and the drains would need to be addressed.

It was like the movie *Groundhog Day*, but I wasn't watching it; I was living it. I was caught in a loop, and I desperately wanted out!

– 5 4 –

Three Strikes, and You're Out!

Six days later, I was back in Dr. Paine's office for another round of post-op appointments. He removed the bandages, checked the stitches and drains, and made sure healing was proceeding as expected. Then he tightly wrapped clean bandages around my chest to keep the swelling down.

I left, praying that this time, he got it right. Admittedly, trusting him after the last surgery was not easy. So when I passed by a mirror, I paused to see if I could tell if the swelling had been reduced.

On June 25, four weeks after the surgery, I went back to see Dr. Paine.

He said, "Well, Evelyn, everything looks good, but let's keep the bandages on to help the swelling go down."

I did, although I was eager to see the final results. *Just be patient; just be patient,* I would tell myself.

Over the next six weeks, though, the pain intensified. It felt like three bowling balls were rolling around on my chest, and the severe and constant cramps under my arm added to my misery.

On August 10, I had another appointment with Dr. Paine. Bob was out of town, so my sister Shirley went with me. I fumed in the examination room while waiting for him to come in to see me. As soon as he entered and asked how I was doing, I responded with all claws exposed.

"Dr. Paine, I am not pleased. I am in *severe* pain. And the three bowling balls on my chest don't help. My chest is so heavy. I feel like I now have three breasts, one on the right, one on the left side of my chest, and one under my left arm. You've placed my left breast so far to the side toward my underarm that I can't lower my left arm all the way down. Is this the way it's supposed to be? I'm miserable. What have I done wrong? What did I ever do to you?"

Shirley calmly yet firmly explained the situation from a medical provider's perspective and that it was not acceptable. He again said he would fix it. He never admitted what he had done to me, but he didn't deny it either.

Undoubtedly, Dr. Paine didn't listen to me . . . had never listened to me. He had his own vision for what my appearance should be with the reconstruction. I should have known when he said, "All women want bigger breasts."

I should not have gotten the reconstruction. Instead, I should have accepted life without breasts. I should have changed doctors, but Bob and I had gone along with Dr. Paine's advice, to be patient and give the swelling time to go down, and when it didn't, we believed he would do the right thing and fix it.

But here we were again. It really brought home the saying, "Fool me once, shame one you. Fool me twice, shame on me."

In other words, no one was to blame but me. I started crying in his office. Shirley put her arm around my shoulder.

"I'll do another surgery," he offered. "This takes time, Evelyn. I'll eventually get it right."

"Eventually?" I repeated, even more devastated by his words. "What do you mean by 'eventually'? I want this done *now!*"

What was happening? Was he trying to deform me? I was so afraid because I knew of women deformed by plastic surgeons who had done breast reconstruction surgeries on them and didn't do it correctly.

Why can't these doctors get it right? Do they have any idea how important it is to these women? Do they care?

I wasn't sure I could believe my doctor anymore because every time I listened to him, I ended up with very bad results. In fact, what he had done to me again was more devastating than the first reconstruction surgery he did. Although I didn't like the way my chest looked after the mastectomy, I was able to cover it up. Now I had two very large breasts of different sizes that couldn't be covered up.

But for this man to keep performing surgery on me, acting so confident, promising me that he would give me just what I wanted, and then getting it grossly wrong over and over was unconscionable. He had traumatized his patient!

So what did I do? I accepted Dr. Paine's offer to do another surgery!

That night, I cried more, blaming myself again. What had I done to my body?

Bob called, and I told him about my appointment with Dr. Paine. "It's all my fault." And I repeated the same should haves, would haves, and could haves that I had been telling myself all day.

"Evie," Bob interrupted. "This is not your fault. It's the doctor's fault. Quit blaming yourself for what he's done."

"I guess you're right," I responded. But I wasn't convinced.

Over the next two months, my situation didn't improve; in fact, it worsened. My body endured a lot of suffering. If I turned the wrong way, the air seemed to be sucked right out of my lungs and would force me to bend over in pain. It was so bad that if anyone was around when this happened, I couldn't even speak to alert them about it.

I was also desperate to get rid of this severe debilitating pain under my left arm. Pain outpowered my anger. So I allowed them to roll me back into surgery to redo the reconstruction and stop what was hurting me so much.

What was I doing? What had I done to myself? How could I have agreed to another surgery with this doctor? I couldn't believe how many surgeries I already had with him, and now, we were doing it again.

Should I stop? I can't stop; the pain is too bad.

I was so confused, exhausted, and in too much pain.

It really didn't come as a surprise that the third surgery by him didn't work either. My breasts were still uneven, and the horrific pain remained.

Sure, it was very disappointing, even devastating. But I was done with Dr. Paine. He was not capable of doing my reconstruction surgery correctly. And for sure, he would never operate on me again!

Well, so I thought . . .

I proved the adage of "Never say never." Eight months later, on June 9, 2016, I was back in Dr. Paine's office. I didn't want to be there, but I was desperate, hoping he would help me. He had started this process, and he was the only plastic surgeon I knew at that time. I was praying he would finally fix his mistakes.

"Dr. Paine," I started, "the skin on my left breast has split. The implants are too big. The implants are *TOO* big. They actually extend under my arm, still making it difficult for my arms to fall naturally at my sides."

His eyes followed everywhere I referred to with no expression.

"Why are they so big when I was very clear I wanted

a small C-cup?" I demanded. I was so frustrated from not being listened to.

"The pain never subsided," I continued. "I experience debilitating nerve pain multiple times a day in my upper side between my breast and my underarm, and I can't move until it subsides."

There was no doubt in my mind that Dr. Paine had to see what I was complaining about.

He responded by saying, "Don't worry, Evelyn, I'll get it right. These things take time."

I thought, *How much time? How many surgeries? What are we talking about here?*

At this point, I truly didn't believe he cared. I was just another widget on his assembly line. He always had one right behind me and one in front of me as we all rode on his conveyor belt waiting for his attention to address our broken pieces. The stories were all the same, but the bodies were all different, the needs were all different, and the goals, what each patient person wanted to achieve, were all different.

This belt led to his indifference, and no one seemed to hold him accountable. While we added emotionally broken to the physically broken and turned our lives upside down, he continued on with his life undeterred.

I wouldn't be surprised if in his mind, he was telling himself, "Some of my work is good, some, well, not so much. Oh, well. My waiting room is packed; my surgery schedule is full. Next!"

– 5 5 –
An Answer to Prayer

After my long and frustrating experience with Dr. Paine, I decided to take a break and give my body time to heal, to see what my breasts looked like when all was said and done.

I still couldn't help second-guessing myself. Should I not have had reconstruction surgery? I didn't know the answer to that question at that time, but what I did know was that I would never go back to Dr. Paine again. He was obviously too busy, and I was tired of being merely a number to him.

I had resigned myself to my condition. I just didn't know what to do. At this point, I had become too skeptical and jaded about plastic surgery, especially for me.

After all, my challenges with the reconstruction surgeries were no secret. It was embarrassing because people were able to see the results as well as my physical pain. However, they weren't able to see the emotional pain it had caused me as well.

Less than two months after my last visit with Dr. Paine (and I mean my *last* visit), my sister Shirley called and told us about a plastic surgeon in in the Jacksonville area, who was referred to her by a friend. "Evie," she said, "his name's Dr. Jonathan Evans, and he's a doctor who listens. My friend said that you would love him!"

Although skeptical, I was also intrigued, not to mention I was still struggling with debilitating pain. Something had to be done to fix the fiasco created by Dr. Paine.

So with great trepidation, I called Dr. Evans's office and made an appointment for August 10. Bob would be home at that time, and he and Shirley would go with me so that they could give their feedback about him, good, bad, or indifferent.

When we walked into Dr. Evans's waiting room, I noticed some differences immediately. First, his staff was kind to me, and his waiting room had no one in it.

Was there something wrong with this doctor? Did no one want to go to him for their plastic surgery needs? Did he not have any other patients? If so, why? Should we stay or go?

I chose to stay and meet with the doctor anyway. After all, we were already there.

Our wait time was very short, which actually added to my concern and convinced me that he couldn't get or keep patients. I couldn't help but wonder why.

The nurse led us to an exam room in the back. I climbed up on the exam table, and Shirley sat in the only chair. Bob stood next to me and held my hand. We all looked around the room, but none of us spoke as we all appeared to be taking everything in.

Then a slim man of medium height with black hair, warm face, and warm eyes walked into the room exuding confidence and holding the medical records I had brought to his office. He welcomed us, and I sensed his words were genuine.

I started telling him about everything, and he focused his gaze on my eyes, glancing down to my chest periodically.

He smiled. "It's going to be okay, Evelyn. I hear you. I have fixed so many patients who have had problems. I can help you too."

I did know that for once, I didn't feel rushed. Instead, I felt as if I was his only patient and that he respected me as his patient, as a person. Therefore, he had set aside this part of his day to focus only on me, which would explain why he didn't have a waiting room full of people. He wanted to take his time to examine me and ask a multitude of questions. Then he repeated back to me my answers.

It was amazing, like I had walked into a dream world where a plastic surgeon cared about his patients and actually listened to them. And he was unbelievably intelligent about his field.

Dr. Evans corroborated my concerns, pointing out problem areas that had been my contention and providing solutions. He even told me how he was going to decrease my cup size to a C, something I had been screaming into the wind with Dr. Paine. This doctor was an answer to my prayers!

Not only did he listen to what I had to say but he had the skill and talent to resolve the problems that had beset me. He told me he could tell immediately that the implants were too large for what I had been wanting. He whole-heartedly agreed that I should not have a breast implant under my arm, especially since it prevented me from placing my arm in a natural position at my side.

He figured out in that first appointment that a pinched nerve was causing the debilitating pain on my left side at the edge of the implant and slightly under my arm. "We'll need to get MRIs to make sure," he stated.

Then he added, "Unfortunately, it's going to take two surgeries to repair the work that has already been done."

My eyes popped open wide. *Oh, dear God! I thought. More surgeries, more surgeries, more surgeries.* Then, *Calm down, Evelyn. God will give you the strength.*

His eyes softened at my look of dismay. He explained, "In the first surgery, I'll need to replace the implants that are already there and reposition them so that you'll no longer feel the weight of bowling balls on your chest. Then in the second surgery, I'll need to repair the area where you have a pinched nerve from the latissimus dorsi flap; it was done incorrectly. I'll do a lot of clean up there as well as redo the scars with better stitching inside and out."

Whew! That made sense.

He went on to explain that he would try to cut through my current incisions to prevent making as few scars as possible. "Still," he said, "there may be some new scars. I'll try my best."

I actually laughed. Scars were just an afterthought by this time. Most important was getting rid of the pain.

Dr. Evans gave me so much hope in that one appointment that all these issues would be resolved and that I would have the last of it behind me. I could go on with my life . . . finally!

At the end of that appointment, which lasted longer than all of my appointments with Dr. Paine combined, we gathered our belongings to leave.

Dr. Evans asked, "May I pray with you before you go?"

Bob and I looked at each other. We both smiled with both joy and relief.

Oh my, I can breathe for the first time in years!

I began to sob with happiness. I wished I had known about Dr. Evans in the beginning. God had given him his talent and gifting and helped him obtain the medical knowledge he would someday need to fix me! *Hallelujah!*

I took his hands, and he prayed. His prayer confirmed that he was the doctor who was going to fix all the pain I had gone through and correct what the other doctor had gotten so wrong. I felt it in my whole body.

Before leaving, I scheduled the first of the two surgeries. The three of us walked to the parking lot to go home, and I felt God's presence walking with us. Although I was nervous and a little afraid about two more surgeries, I felt confident that they would be the last. After all this time, what more could I ask for?

And I was not disappointed!

The two surgeries that Dr. Evans did on me were not as painful as the ones with Dr. Paine. He had such a kind and gentle bedside manner from the moment we met to just before falling asleep before the surgeries and throughout all my post-op visits. The differences between him and Dr. Paine couldn't have been greater.

As I healed, the swelling decreased just like I had thought it should. The bowling balls, the debilitating pain that had knocked me to my knees from Dr. Paine's past surgeries, the large breasts, all gone!

Sadly, I had gotten to the point where all I knew was pain, so not having it anymore was actually a wonderful and blessed new normal that I had to get used to (yes, I had to get used to not having pain). But no worries, I got used to it quickly! It was as if God had performed a miracle, and I now had the beautiful breasts I had been wanting.

Because of one doctor, I was a physical and emotional wreck. But then, because of another doctor, I now live a pain-free life. Dr. Evans knew enough, studied enough, and loved his job enough to do it right. So many women who go through these surgeries with bad doctors can't afford to get them fixed because of insurance and because the doctors don't really care.

I was blessed by God to have been told about Dr. Evans. Finally, a plastic surgeon who listened, and as a result, he changed my life. Shirley's friend was right—*I did love him!*

We learned not to judge a book by its cover, or in this situation, by how many people sat in a waiting room. For a plastic surgeon, having a packed waiting room wasn't always a good sign. However, Dr. Evans focused on one patient at a time, making sure that he gave them the attention they deserved. He was a doctor who cared about the individual more than the number of individuals.

We all want to trust our doctors, but sometimes, we get dealt a doctor who doesn't listen and perform well. If we had come to this man first, it would have saved me a whole year of misery and let me get back to living a normal life a whole year sooner. Lesson learned—do my due diligence and don't settle.

Dr. Jonathan Evans played a huge role in my getting my life back, and I'll be forever grateful to him. But it was more than that. Because I was able to finally get my life back, Bob and I were able to get our life together back!

We were not and are not anything special, at least not to this world. We've never strived to be because we take comfort in knowing that we are very special to our Lord and Savior Jesus Christ. If not for Him, I wouldn't be here telling you our story and testimony. And if not for Him, we wouldn't be two cancer victims turned survivors turned victors!

−56−

Conclusion

Our story is one of love, one of faith, one of miracles, and one of grace and mercy. Cancer tried to destroy Bob and me one by one, but with God's protection, healing took place one by one. Bob started first and then held my hand and heart until I caught up. Every step of the way, God used love and humor as the glue that held us together and carried us as one set of footprints.

Bob's ten-year mark was November 2021, and I hit my five-year mark in June 2018. My ten-year mark is right around the corner—June 2023. And we're still going doubly strong like two layers of steel.

To anyone who doesn't know our story, we appear to be a loving couple who hasn't experienced any worries and concerns. And they would be right to a certain degree! Sure, we have worries and concerns just like the next person, but when cancer attacked us, we fought back on our knees so that we could put it at the foot of the cross. When there, it had to contend with a powerful three-string cord: Bob, me, and God! Cancer never had a chance.

So all of cancer's attempts backfired in a big way. It's supposed to cause weakness, but instead, it gave us strength. We plowed right through it and beyond. Bob ended up proving the doctors wrong; he was able to return to his active lifestyle, including surfing. As strangers joined me on the beach one day to cheer him on after he had paddled out with one arm, jumped up on his board, and then beautifully surfed a wave, tears of joy and thankfulness came to my eyes.

Granted, Bob is physically limited to some degree, but we're here to tell you that living with side effects is better than not living at all. Knowing what he was forced to endure due to neck and throat cancer makes it more miraculous. He proved that it's not about someone being unable to do something ever again; it's about how motivated they are to make it happen. Adaptation is not a cop out; it's an opt in. The way Bob keeps all that's dear to him is not focusing on what was but what can be. With this new normal, he looks at everything differently, savoring it all a little more than ever before.

As for me, I had thought that all the physical changes I had undergone on the outside would change me, Evelyn Kormondy, on the inside. At first, I found them shocking, but they didn't shock my husband, and they sure didn't shock God. And everyone else seemed to accept them too, even embrace them. So I learned to roll with the punches and accepted them as well. It didn't mean that the changes were bad, just different. More importantly, they were evidence of my healing. After all, if cancer couldn't beat me, then neither could these changes.

But our journeys through cancer would have been different if not for our wonderful support team—our family, friends, and church family. They were always there, answering our cries in times of need. If not for them, the challenge would have been so much more difficult. Everything they did was appreciated more than they could fathom!

As a result, I pray that there will always be someone to help a cancer patient. This help can come with your time, such as taking the patient to a medical appointment, getting them groceries, picking up their medication, doing their laundry, cleaning their house, praying with them, or simply making them laugh. Any type of help and assistance is treasured. For those who can help financially, any amount would be appreciated as well.

If nothing else, cancer victims could use your encouragement. Unfortunately, cancer is not limited to a physical illness that's contended with on a physical level; it affects its victim mentally as well, so the battle also takes place in the mind to stay strong. Anything you can do to help them stay strong would go beyond being appreciated.

If you're the one struggling with cancer, you can make it through it with God's love and help and with the love of others around you. You are not a diagnosis!

Today, our lives are perfect and filled with joy. Are they the same as before? No, they are so much more. The deep walk with God has filled every part of our bodies and souls with the beauty of all that's around us, especially with the kind people we've met along the way. Many were meant to be in our lives only for a short time. We won't ever see them again, but we'll never forget them. Some of them remain friends for life. They continue to lift our spirits, make us smile, make us laugh, and even cry with us.

Before cancer tried to have its way with Bob and me, we didn't think our faith could get any stronger than it was, but oh, how wrong we were! Through our journey, we've learned that faith and love have no depth nor width nor height. It is and has been without boundaries, and for this, we are very thankful!

Inspirational Poems

—By Peggy Dailey—

Burnt

The pain is great
The burning ongoing
As the radiation beam hones in
On the cancer within

No escape available
To leave this time
Hope is dashed
The burn numbs the mind

The will to live carries her thru
A vision of joy and good health anew
And so she marches on each day
Praying this truly is the way

Out of this sorrow so great
Sometimes feeling the cancer berets
The safety of her heartfelt faith
Believing she always will escape

Just like the skin she sheds with such pain
She is determined to rise again
Renewed, reborn to live on
For now we must keep her encircled
safely in our arms

Lifting prayers to God above
To continue to shower her with love
Strength to endure the now
So she can have a future
that will be a wonderful wow!

Fatigue

Fatigue can defeat you
Make it impossible to get up and go
Eating, drinking, smiling are such an effort
A not-so-simple task for those who know

That the constant barrage of questions and pain
Drive you deeper into your brain
Making it difficult to greet the day
Wearing you out as the daytime remains

It is then that you are entitled to shout,
"Everyone get out!
Let me sleep and regroup!
Forget about the homemade soup!"

With the grace of those who love you and wait
Hoping that when you wake
Fatigue has exited this space
And once again you are in this race

Speeding down the road long
Held up by those who mourn
Because of your pain and difficult task
Always believing it will pass

So when you are fatigued and need to rest
Lean on me, I'll help you with your task
The battle royale – hard it is true
And bring you to victory
with the gratitude of more than just a few!

Hair

It's there, it's there I see her hair
Growing up everywhere
No more shiny scalp
Just hair all about

A victory of sorts
Past the chemo and the pain
Beyond the radiation burn
Seeing herself and her beginning mane

Time will tell where it will go
Moving on to joy and less woe
Starting to look more like herself
A true warrior fighting on

A joyous lilt in her voice has returned
Her bright smile and her hugging arms
Happiness rings out for all to hear
Sorely missed for the past year

Where this will go, I don't know
But let's just sit back and watch the hair grow
Up towards heaven
and Our Heavenly Father's throne
He always reminds her she was never alone

To victory and such
We send lots of hugs
Waiting with anticipation
Will she make it pink
or a multi-colored configuration?

It's Personal

She battles this killer alone
Even with many of them in the room
Holding to her, not letting go
But even though they know

She is the only one now
Who feels the pain all around
And struggles every day to smile
Trying to forget for a while

How fleeting a life's day can be
As this killer tries to steal her you see
Snuff out the light, silence the laugh
Bringing down the shade

It is personal, this battle royale
No one but she can lead the chase
Making it exit her body, her space
While we all stand and see
the pain on her face

The poison is dripping
Wiping out the good and the bad
Leaving destruction in its path
Hopefully this cure will last

And with the dawning of a future day
We can hold her up as she makes her way
Carefully, so weak with the pain
Hoping all this leads to a big gain

Starting over, leaving the past
To a new start that will last
And then her smile will return
As we give thanks for all we learned

The human spirit is stronger than
Any disease that tried to end
A bright life, a dancing friend
Leaving behind the sorrow. AMEN!

Joy-Filled News

The news was spoken matter-of-factly
As if it was another comment for the day
Her cancer has finally gone away
She if free to run and play

Left scarred and injured, true
But these too will pass away
She will return to laugh and smile
Her bravery shining all the while

We must still hold her close
In our hearts and prayers
As she makes her way forward
To the life she fought so hard to keep

I see her smile has returned
Her laugh is renewing
And now she plans for her future
All the while reviewing

What has happened in this past year
Only a warrior could survive
Shouldering all the pain and suffering
With great hopefulness all the while

So let us rejoice and sing praise
Dearest Evelyn has survived
And may her future be long and bright
Giving praise and thanksgiving
to God all the while

Free again
Free again
Praise be to God
Evelyn is free again!

Pink Ribbons

She stood lost in the abyss
Gazing at herself in the looking glass
She never thought that she would miss
The soft tissue mass that formed her breast

And then she saw it, the pink ribbon
Soft and flowing, hanging from her chair
She wondered how many others wore it
To show the world in hope we are united

This battle, it is long and at times hard
But then you remember
the beautiful flowers in the yard
That bear testament life is a constant blooming
And on the horizon a new day is looming

With it will come the love and the care
Knowing the pink ribbons we all will wear
To tell the hurting sisters of the family of man
You are not forgotten, together we take a stand

And in the not-too-distant future you will see
Breast cancer disappear
from the lives of you and me

With love, Peggy Dailey

Toxic

The doctor's visit was long
The sad tale was spawned
No more chemo for her
The destruction to her body profound

Battered and beaten down
The poison swam around
Destroying veins and toes and feet
Unable to walk safely around

Now the surgery must move up
The tumor is growing—it is tough
Weak and worn, her body cannot fight
Fear is she will not have the reserve to survive

She is writing her letters of goodbye
Checking her will to ensure
They all know her love is true
What else can she do?

Fearfully she will go
If they can find space on the O.R. schedule time
And as she closes her eyes to start the feat
She worries that when she opens them,
the angels she will meet

Inspirational Scriptures

FOR GOING THROUGH TRIALS AND TRIBULATIONS

Peace I leave with you; my peace I give you. I do not give to you as the world gives. Do not let your hearts be troubled and do not be afraid.

~John 14:27 NIV~

Praise the LORD, my soul, and forget not all his benefits who forgives all your sins and heals all your diseases, who redeems your life from the pit and crowns you with love and compassion.

~Psalms 103:2–4 NIV~

The LORD is my shepherd, I lack nothing.

He makes me lie down in green pastures,

he leads me beside quiet waters,

he refreshes my soul.

He guides me along the right paths

for his name's sake.

Even though I walk

through the darkest valley,

I will fear no evil,

for you are with me;

your rod and your staff,

they comfort me.

You prepare a table before me

in the presence of my enemies.

You anoint my head with oil;

my cup overflows.

Surely your goodness and love will follow me

all the days of my life,

and I will dwell in the house of the LORD

forever."

~Psalm 23 NIV~

Let all that you do be done in love.

~1 Corinthians 16:14 ASV~

Anyone who does not love does not know God, because **God is love**.

~1 John 4:8 ESV~

And above all these put on love, which binds everything together in perfect harmony.

~Colossians 3:14 ESV~

A new commandment I give to you, that you love one another: just as I have loved you, you also are to love one another. By this all people will know that you are my disciples, if you have love for one another.

~John 13:34–35 ESV~

Love is patient, love is kind. It does not envy, it does not boast, it is not proud. It does not dishonor others, it is not self-seeking, it is not easily angered, it keeps no record of wrongs. Love does not delight in evil but rejoices with the truth. It always protects, always trusts, always hopes, always perseveres. Love never fails . . .

~1 Corinthians 13:4–8 NIV~

If my people, who are called by my name, will humble themselves and pray and seek my face and turn from their wicked ways, then I will hear from heaven, and I will forgive their sin and will heal their land. Now my eyes will be open and my ears attentive to the prayers offered in this place.

~2 Chronicles 7:14–15 NIV~

Helpful Hints

The following are some helpful hints I want to give you if you or a loved one is diagnosed with cancer:

- Make a list of questions for your doctors. Then ask him or her:

  ◦ Can I record the answers? (Otherwise, you'll have trouble remembering things because there is so much to take in.)

  ◦ What additional tests are needed to be performed prior to surgery?

  ◦ When can we schedule such tests and expect the results?

  ◦ What is recommended as far as the surgery and the recovery time?

  ◦ Will there be additional surgeries needed? If yes, for what?

◦ What type of treatments do you recommend? Please explain the treatments, side effects, duration, frequency, etc.

◦ When will treatments begin?

◦ Is there anything I can do to prepare myself for this journey, such as exercise, diet, stretching?

◦ Are there organizations I need to be in contact with to help?

◦ Will I be assigned a social worker to help?

- Get a three-ring binder and keep all information in it to refer back to.
- Please try and stay away from sugar. Prevention prevents pain.
- Know that it's okay to let your body rest. And, it's okay to let others help you.

About the Author

—Evelyn Kormondy—

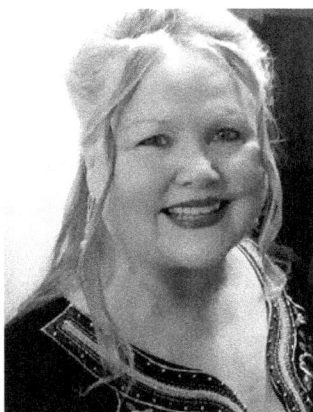

Born into a family of six girls, Evelyn grew up a self-proclaimed Daddy's girl. She worked for his company, Ashcroft Creative Cabinets, where she was an interior designer, accountant, and secretary for eighteen years. Toward the end of her time at Ashcroft's, she also worked as a weekend hostess in a restaurant. Not only did she earn supplemental income while there, but she also met Bob, the love of her life.

In 1996, she went back to school to be trained as a neuromuscular therapist and received her massage therapy license a year later. In 2001, she "retired" to become a full-time domestic engineer so that she could be there for Bob when he was home as well as free up her schedule to travel with him.

However, Evelyn isn't one to let grass grow under her feet. With a husband who is a cameraman for major sports events and recipient of six Emmy Awards, getting into photography was bound to happen. After all, she had the best teacher. In 2010, she took her new skill and passion for nature and sports and became a professional photographer, shooting pictures for various magazines.

Then cancer turned their lives upside down.

Since her recovery from cancer, she has reclaimed some parts of her life while other parts have been created. Thankful to her Lord and Savior Jesus Christ for giving her and Bob a second chance, she gives back by volunteering at her church's food pantry to feed the needy, coordinating a team of sixty-six volunteers.

Her second chance has also increased her passion for having friends over and cooking for them and her love for her big family. She's most proud of her roles as stepmother/bonus mom to three amazing girls and as aunt, great-aunt, and great great-aunt.

In the midst of her busy life, she and Bob still travel the world together for his different assignments and make new memories to add to their collection. In fact, there's nothing she enjoys more than spending time with her two favorite men—her daddy and her husband—the love of her life!

For Evelyn Kormondy, she's still living the dream, but this time around, she takes time to smell the roses and to touch someone else's life along the way.

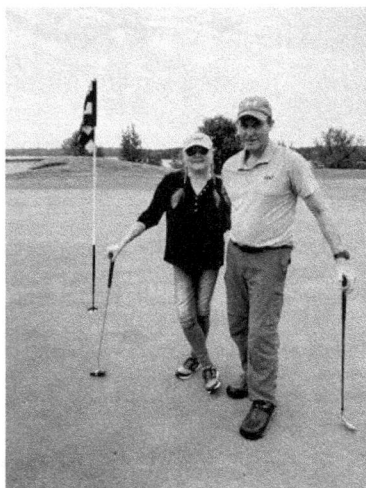

*Back to work the Celebrity Golf
Tournament Lake Tahoe*

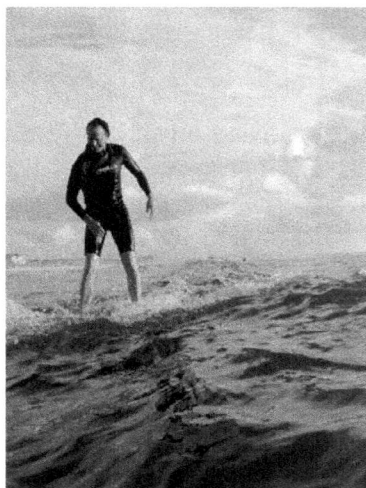

*Catching a wave for the
first time with God*

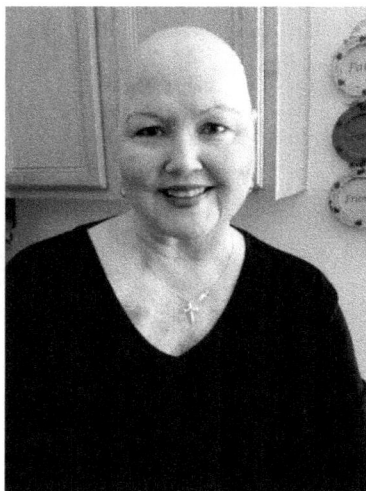

*Feeling pretty
rocking the bald*

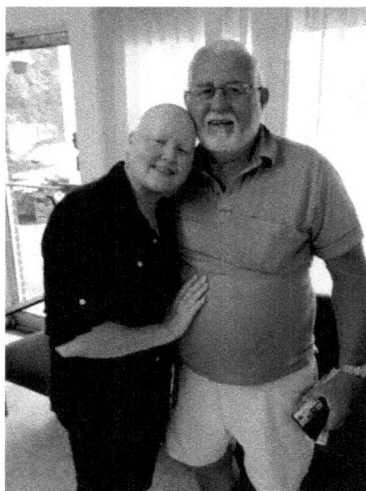

*Daddy taking his little girl
to the barbershop*

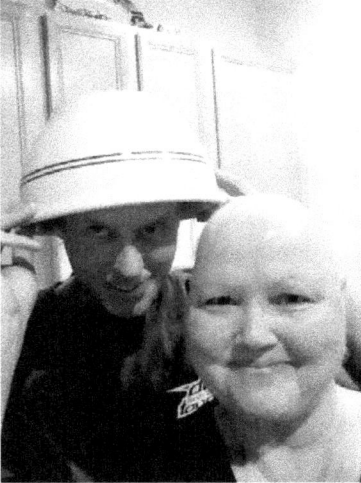

*Embracing the moment of being
bald with the one you love*

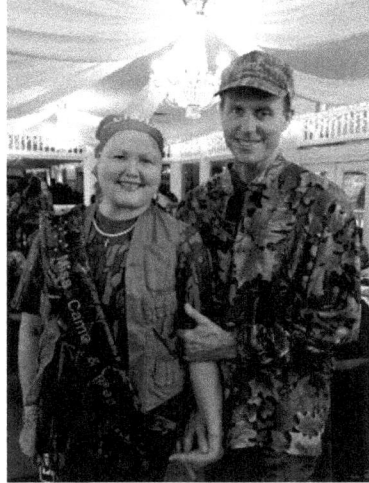

*Feeling special at
Camo & Pearls*

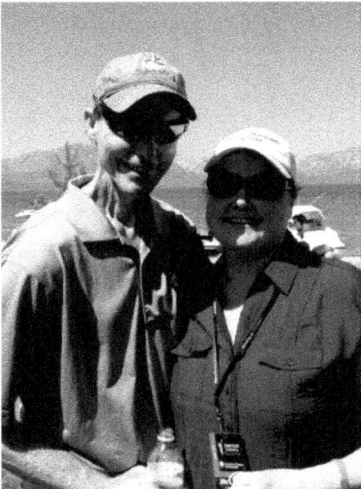

*Enjoying life
after our battle*

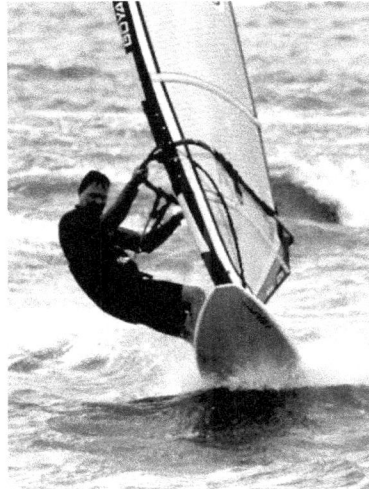

*Very fortunate to be
able to windsurf*

www.ingramcontent.com/pod-product-compliance
Lightning Source LLC
Chambersburg PA
CBHW060304030426
42336CB00011B/932